The Practice of
Primary Nursing

Printing and Binding by Eyre & Spottiswoode Ltd, London and Margate

THE PRACTICE OF

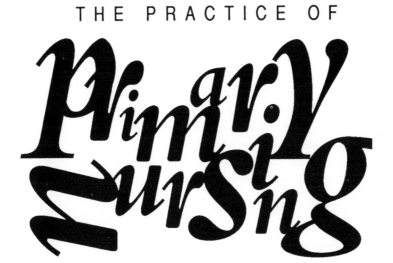

PRIMARY NURSING

MARIE MANTHEY RN MNA

Published by the King's Fund Centre
126 Albert Street
London
NW1 7NF

Tel: 071 267 6111

ISBN 1 85717 017 2

A CIP catalogue record for this book is available from the British Library

Distributed by Bournemouth English Book Centre (BEBC)
9 Albion Close
Parkstone
Poole
Dorset
BH12 3LL

The King's Fund Centre is a health services development agency which promotes
improvements in health and social care. We do this by working with people in
health services, in social services, in voluntary agencies, and with the users of their
services. We encourage people to try out new ideas, provide financial or practical
support to new developments, and enable experiences to be shared through
workshops, conferences and publications. Our aim is to ensure that good
developments in health and social care are widely taken up.

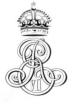

The King's Fund Centre is a part of the
King Edward's Hospital Fund for London.

CONTENTS

FOREWORD

When this book was published in 1980, Primary Nursing had been around long enough in the United States to have acquired some external trappings that this publication helped to dispel. There is something about Primary Nursing that appeals to the highest consciousness nurses have about their profession. And it is an easy step from considering the potential provided by Primary Nursing to wanting to achieve 'perfect nursing'. However, 'perfect nursing' is usually linked to a level of staffing seldom achieved in the real world. So, when this book was published, one of the major myths to be debunked was that staffing levels and Primary Nursing correlated. Primary Nursing can work well when staffing is short and doesn't automatically work well when staffing is adequate.

Another 'trapping' was the idea that it could be implemented by management edict or, on the other hand, in the absence of administrative support. Neither alternative is successful, and this book helps explain, in simple language, why not.

The text of this edition has been changed to reflect British spelling and grammar but the only substantive change in content reflects a change in my position. When this book was written, I had occasionally used exceptional LPNs (the equivalent of an enrolled nurse) as Primary Nurses. As experience with the system moved throughout the United States and as our understanding of the role in relationship to licensure grew, it became apparent that this was not an acceptable use of LPNs. The situation now is such that there is a national consensus this role is reserved for registered nurses in acute care hospitals. LPNs do function as Primary Nurses in long-term care situations.

One of the major changes this type of nursing generates is in the role of the ward sister or charge nurse. We found in the United States that individuals in that role (often called head nurse or nurse manager) had to learn new skills. In fact, the whole management structure needs to adjust to the idea of decentralised decision making. Professional practice at the bedside is based on the concept of recognising the legitimate authority of the staff nurse to make decisions about the patient's care. Chapter five outlines these issues that are so important to creating the appropriate atmosphere for the risk-taking of professional practice.

I am delighted to write this foreword for the book's publication in Great Britain. One of the greatest sources of the strength of nursing is the universal values we share. I trust the readers of this edition will find those values in abundance in this book and in your practice.

Marie Manthey
Creative Nursing Management
January 1992

FOREWORD

Some years ago, when I first became interested in primary nursing, I heard the name Marie Manthey mentioned and started to hunt for her book. It had been recommended to me as 'essential reading' but trying to track it down proved far more difficult than I would have believed. Imagine my dismay when I discovered that it was no longer available in the United Kingdom. However, not to be defeated, I eventually tracked down some copies which had been hidden away in a warehouse and the effort proved well worth while. If people wanted a simple, straightforward and practical guide to primary nursing this was the text for them.

As more and more people became interested in the subject I found that my own copy was almost permanently on loan. Wide reference was made to the work by many other authors but actually getting hold of the original work remained problematic. However, it was not until last year that I first met Marie and had the opportunity to talk more with her about her ideas and the possibility of republishing her book in the UK.

There is no doubt that Marie's work has stood the test of time. While, in her very practical way, she has continued to develop the advice she offers in relationship to implementing primary nursing, the principles have remained the same. The work is practical and easy to read, despite the complex issues which are discussed. Minor adjustments have been made to make it more applicable to the British reader but the greater part of the work stands as it was first written. Maybe it is because the origin of the ideas arose from practice nurses themselves seeking more satisfactory ways of managing their day-to-day work that it is so accessible — for it tells the story of why they choose to change their way of practice in the first place. Thus it becomes clear that the roots of primary nursing do not lie in a theoretical idea which was imposed on practice, but on a practical solution to an everyday work problem generated by the pactitioners themselves.

Marie herself has concern that primary nursing will be 'imposed', despite her commitment to the principles on which it is founded. Without a clear understanding of why the changes may be beneficial and what the implications are for both practitioners and those they work with much would be lost. Reading this text makes clear why, and how, one group of nurses chose to change their approach and may be helpful to many more in clarifying their own ideas.

Despite the plethora of British work which has arisen in relation to primary nursing over the last decade, this book still has an important contribution to make. Many people have taken the original ideas and described and developed them. However, returning to the source work offers British nurses an opportunity to hear about primary nursing, as it was originally described, in order that they can interpret it in their own way.

So it is with great delight that we have taken the opportunity of making this text readily available in the UK. I hope you will find it as helpful as I have over the years.

Barbara Vaughan
Director, Nursing Development Unit
King's Fund Centre
January 1992

PREFACE

This book is written for anyone who wants to know about Primary Nursing. It is not meant to be the last word on the subject, nor is it the first. I have tried to be clear in writing about this system, because the system itself is very simple. However, because it is not also easy, there is a tendency to make it seem more complex than it is. In my efforts to honour the beauty of its simplicity, some may feel I have ignored or slighted important complex related issues. I prefer to err in favour of simplicity, but have tried to deal thoroughly with every issue of *immediate importance to the system*. If there are complex issues I have not dealt with adequately in this book it is because I do not feel they are central to Primary Nursing. Everything is related to everything else in this world, so lines have to be drawn and mine have been drawn rather tightly around the system of Primary Nursing.

Primary Nursing is a delivery system designed: 1) to allocate 24-hour responsibility for each patient's care to one individual nurse, and 2) to assign this nurse the actual provision of her patient's physical care whenever possible. The Primary Nurse leaves information and instructions for her patient's care when she is off duty, so the nurse who relieves her knows about the patient as a person and exactly how care should be administered in this particular case. The Primary Nurse also has major responsibility for preparing the patient and/or his family for discharge.

Primary Nursing is a system for delivering nursing care in an inpatient facility; that is *all* it is. It is not a solution to the problem of the difference between 'professional' and 'technical' levels of practice and preparation; it is not a solution to the issues created by the use of licensed practical nurses (LPNs) in acute care settings. It will not solve staffing problems caused by an inadequate budget, nor will it increase the workload. (So budgets should not be expanded in the name of Primary Nursing!) It will solve neither personnel management nor interpersonal relationship problems. It is a system originally designed for delivering nursing care to sick people who are hospitalised. It was developed on a real station in a real hospital during a period of serious nurse-power shortage. The staff was not hand-picked, nor was it considered unusually qualified. Thus, the system is designed for maximum use of *available* resources. No additional monies were allocated from any source during the development phase. It is an innovation that works in the real world because that is the crucible in which it was originally developed and tested.

High quality nursing care should be the goal of every nurse, educator and manager. High quality nursing to me means care that is individualised to a particular patient, administered humanely and competently, comprehensively and with continuity. Primary Nursing is one means of accomplishing that quality of care. It may not be the only way to do so; it is the proven way with which this book concerns itself.

The first part of the book (Chapters One and Two) explains the recent history of nursing in the United States as I understand it to have impacted on the present. I have started with a historical analysis because during ten years of teaching nurses about this system the historical approach has proved to be the most effective way to prepare them to receive the new information with a minimum of rejection. An understanding of how we got where we are helps people avoid becoming defensive about their current situations and opens them to forward motion or a growth experience. To understand why Primary Nursing was developed in the first place, it has been helpful to describe, graphically at times, the problems staff nurses, patients and others experience in using other delivery systems, notably 'team nursing'. Since many people are still struggling mightily to make team nursing work, an understanding of its development from a historical perspective reduces the emotional negativism such a critique can cause.

Primary Nursing evolved from an effort to improve on the implementation of team nursing so that high quality nursing could be effectively achieved. The problems with team nursing as they were experienced in that setting were identified and attempts were made to correct those problems without changing the system. Those efforts failed, so an alternative delivery system was designed. That system was called Primary Nursing. The three problems identified with team nursing were: 1) fragmentation of care; 2) complex channels of communication; and 3) shared responsibility. Recognition of these in turn provided the bases of Primary Nursing. Thus the basic elements, the strengths of Primary Nursing, as described in Chapter Three, are the result of growth and learning from team nursing.

Chapter Four, The Implementation of Primary Nursing, is the backbone of this book. In this chapter I have tried to explain how to implement this system successfully based on all the experience I have had doing so in the past ten years. The recommendations for implementation which I make are a result of what I learned as I implemented the concept and what I learned from the efforts of others using different approaches.

My observations and conclusions are a product of my values and beliefs about mankind. I am an equalitarian with strong anti-elitist prejudices. I believe that mankind and womankind are good and that people want to do the right thing; thus, I have a great deal of confidence in the integrity of a system designed by the staff members who will use it. I truly believe that a system so implemented will provide an effective way to deliver high quality care. Thus, my recommendations about implementation focus intensely on staff member involvement in the implementation process.

Rehumanisation of hospital care is the goal that has been my strongest motivation. Decentralised decision making seems to me to be the organisational framework within which humane treatment of the sick can most effectively be provided and maintained. In order for the patient to be treated humanely, the staff who deliver the care must be treated humanely by the management of the institution. Decentralised decision making is an organisational framework wherein authority for decision making is delegated downwards in the institution to the level of action which, in nursing, is the bedside. By authorising the staff, who deliver care, to decide how that care will be delivered, the institution recognises that the staff are intelligent and educated human beings whose intellects can be used in deciding how to provide sensitive and sensible individualised care. Decentralised decision making recognises the inherent worth of the intelligence each employee can bring to care of the patients. Patients cannot receive humane and thoughtful care from staff members who have been treated in a dehumanised fashion by their managers.

Management responsibilities in a decentralised decision-making structure are clearly different from those in a centralised, authoritarian structure. One of the most obvious differences is that the thrust of management in a decentralised setting is facilitative rather than directive. In Primary Nursing implementation, the change process should be dominated by the staff nurses. The decision to put the Primary Nursing system into effect must be made at the staff nurse level. Otherwise, decentralised decision making has not been experienced by the staff nurses and cannot be successfully used in the clinical decision making required by the system.

Occasionally, staff nurses resent this implementation style. As a director of nursing I have had staff nurses beg me to tell them what to do, but these are a very small minority of very immature people (of all ages). Most staff nurses eagerly accept the challenge of self-determination and the resulting growth experiences are thrilling to see and profound to feel.

This approach to implementation reflects my deep belief that it is time for nursing to grow up and for staff nurses to stop acting like and being treated like little children. Most staff nurses I have met are mature people. Many have dealt with significant life events and accept heavy life responsibilities. Yet, at work, they are called 'girls', treated like children and made to feel like 'just a staff nurse' (a phrase that is sickeningly similar to 'just a housewife'). The implementation process I recommend gives all staff members an opportunity to use legitimately rights they have always possessed but seldom felt free to use openly.

Nurses need to develop an appreciation for the reality of legitimate authority. Many nurses have been made to feel that because the physician controls medical treatment and the hospital administrator defines the mission and policies of the hospital that these two traditionally male dominated functions also have authority and control over all aspects of nursing practice. If a director of nursing is to be held liable for the quality of care that is administered by the nursing staff, she must have authority to set the standards of care and introduce appropriate delivery systems. This *authority* is legitimately hers by virtue of the *responsibility* she has accepted.

Many directors have asked me how I got the physicians or the hospital administrator to let me do Primary Nursing. The simplest and most honest answer is 'I didn't ask them; I told them'. Since Primary Nursing usually does not cost any more money in salaries, permission, so to speak, from the hospital administrator is not necessary. However, in introducing the concept it is extremely important that all key members of the institution understand the changes being made. In so informing them, however, the director of nursing needs to be aware of the fact that neither the physicians nor the administrator have legitimate authority to tell her what nursing system is appropriate for the nursing staff to use. If that were their job, they could save the cost of the director's salary.

This book is about Primary Nursing—how it developed, what it is and how to implement it. It is also a book about power, self-determination and the humanisation of hospital care. Primary Nursing is not really a new idea. It is a logical approach to caring for sick people the way we would like to be cared for if *we* were sick. However, the process of returning to these simple values is revolutionary in that it represents a reallocation of power—from a faceless, anonymous, hierarchical, authoritarian bureaucracy to the staff nurse who is responsible for the care of a sick person.

It should be noted that staff nurses have been referred to throughout the text as 'she' and sick persons as 'he'. The use of the feminine pronoun for nurses comes easily and naturally, but even though I am proud that nursing has historically been a woman's profession I have not intentionally discriminated against male colleagues. The she/he nurse/patient pairing is simply a matter of convenience adopted purely for the sake of the reader.

ACKNOWLEDGEMENTS

The number of people whose help in preparing this book should really be acknowledged is boundless. Ever since Primary Nursing was first implemented I have had innumerable opportunities to meet and talk with nurses all over the country and from each I have learned and grown.

A special expression of gratitude to those members of the administration of the University of Minnesota Hospitals who, not without taking considerable risks, provided the fertile environment in which Primary Nursing was first developed. John Westerman, Hospital Administrator, and Florence Julian, Director of Nursing, were especially supportive, as was my partner in heading the pilot project, David Preston, and the first head nurse, Diane Bartels. Needless to say, the encouragement and support of the entire nursing staff was both invaluable and appreciated beyond measure.

I would like to thank my typist, Pat Moore, for help of a more concrete nature, and my children Claire and Mark, for help of a more subtle nature. They have helped and supported me at crucial points in my development and I can only hope that I have similarly helped them.

This book is dedicated to Florence Marie Fisher, a nurse who cared for me when I was hospitalised at the age of five with scarlet fever, in St Joseph's Hospital Chicago. Although I never saw her again, her personalised and very humane care of me became a model I have followed throughout my life and professional career. This dedication is also made to all those nurses who recognise the profound influence this special kind of nursing practice can have on the lives of their patients and who, by practising it themselves, perpetuate the proud tradition and invaluable legacy of all of the nurses like Ms Fisher—ultimately the highest tribute of all.

1

THE DEPROFESSIONALISATION OF NURSING

Primary Nursing is a delivery system for nursing at the station level that facilitates professional nursing practice despite the bureaucratic nature of hospitals. The practice of any profession is based on an independent assessment of a client's needs which determines the kind and amount of service to be rendered: services in bureaucracies are usually delivered according to routine pre-established procedures without sensitivity to variations in needs. In bureaucracies, functions are grouped into bureaus or departments, headed by chiefs who usually retain decision-making authority. Thus, for professionals to exist in a bureaucracy, the system used to deliver the services must be designed to minimise the bureaucratic impact and maximise the value of their individualised services.

Within a bureaucracy, many different delivery systems may co-exist to accomplish the many different functions of the various departments. These systems can enhance and facilitate either bureaucratic or professional values depending on the nature of the services rendered and the design of the system. Before Primary Nursing was established at the University of Minnesota in 1969, the delivery system used for hospital nursing reflected bureaucratic rather than professional values. Both functional nursing (in which one nurse passes all medications, another does all treatments and several people give baths) and the team nursing systems are designed according to a mass production model of service delivery; the least complex tasks are assigned to the least trained workers, the more complex to more skilled workers and so on up a hierarchy of task complexity. In those systems, registered nurses are assigned two functions: 1) to administer the most complex tasks and 2) to coordinate and supervise the tasks done by the lesser prepared workers. Registered nurses in these systems are not professional care givers; rather they are checker-uppers of cheaper-doers. Primary Nursing is a delivery system that creates the opportunity for nurses to develop a truly professional role in hospital nursing today.

Seventy years ago, when graduate nurses worked in their patients' own homes, there was no need to be concerned about a delivery system for individualised patient care. The nurse took care of the sick person from the time the need for care was identified until it no longer existed; care was personally administered by the nurse according to the assessment she made of the individual needs of the patient. There were no rules or regulations, no routine procedures, no hospital policies, time schedules, or supervisors. She practised nursing with a degree of independence unheard of in modern hospital nursing.

This type of practice had more of the characteristics sociologists use in describing a profession than does the practice of the modern nurse. It is my contention that despite all the lip service that has been paid to the process of professionalisation, nursing has in fact undergone a serious process of *depro-fessionalisation*. The change in setting from home to hospital and to the delivery systems subsequently designed for the hospital setting have significantly decreased the professionalism of nursing practice.

During those same 70 years, nurse leaders have laboured heroically to upgrade nursing education in the firm belief that higher educational standards elevate professional stature. They changed the setting of education from the hospital, with its apprenticeship training programmes, to the college and its classroom programmes. Their efforts were successful. The majority of nurse preparation now takes place in educational rather than service settings. It is unfortunate however that the effect of that success on nursing's professional stature has been diminished by the simultaneous deprofessionalisation of nursing practice. Primary Nursing is a delivery system that promises to maximise the professional values acquired in these educational programmes by facilitating professional role development.

There are four characteristics generally agreed to by sociologists as descriptive of the ways a profession can be differentiated from another endeavour or occupation. These are: 1) an identifiable body of knowledge that can best be transmitted in a formal educational programme; 2) autonomy of decision making; 3) peer review of practice; and 4) identification with a professional organisation as the standard setter and arbiter of practice. I believe that the practice of nurses in the 1920s contained more of all these characteristics than did the practice of nurses in the 1970s, and that this change in the degree of professionalism is directly attributable to the change in the setting of practice that has occurred over the last seventy years.

A comparison of nursing in the 1920s and the 1970s in terms of the four characteristics of a profession illustrates this point.

The *identifiable body of knowledge* that could best be communicated in a formal educational setting was more clearly identifiable in the 1920s when Nightingale's *Notes on Nursing* was the basic textbook. Today's variety of generic curriculum theories boggles the mind. Different schools teach nursing using different theoretical frameworks and different skill levels, resulting in confusion and ambiguity about what can be expected of graduate nurses. In the 1920s, it was simple; all graduates could fill all nursing needs for all patients! Today, two-year, three-year, and four-year programmes prepare nurses to perform different functions with varying levels of competence in ability to make clinical judgments. While the quality of education is undoubtedly superior now, the confusion and ambiguity over the content has so seriously blurred the boundaries of the body of knowledge that it is no longer clearly identifiable.

Autonomy of decision making is a natural result of acquiring an identifiable body of knowledge, since it follows logically that only those who have acquired this knowledge are qualified to make decisions in that particular field of endeavour. The privilege of decision-making autonomy is based on a clear demarcation of the boundaries of knowledge. Currently, there is much confusion over what nurses know and can do independently. Neither nurses, their patients, nor their colleagues agree about which decisions are appropriately made by a nurse and only a nurse.

In the 1920s, the nurse was concerned with the comfort and treatment of the patient and with maintaining the health of the family. The private duty nurse entered the patient's home and took charge of the patient's total care. There was no head nurse to supervise her and no clinical instructor to orient her. She had the authority to decide when and how the physician's treatment orders were carried out. In addition, she educated her patient and the family about measures they could employ to maintain their own health. It was well understood that during a nurse's stay with a family, she would teach members of the household housekeeping methods, germ theory, comprehensive sanitation techniques, and principles of good nutrition and basic health maintenance. These were part of the nurse's defined body of knowledge. She did not expect, nor was she expected, to consult with the physician or anyone else about routine comfort, sanitation, or nutrition.

In addition, the nurse was the community health educator, in competition with no one else for that role. Nurses, especially public health nurses, were often asked to deliver speeches to community civic groups on topics related to care of the sick and maintenance of health. Graduate nurses were taught how to organise material for a speech and how to deliver a public address, both to a live audience as well as over the radio.

This lack of a clearly defined knowledge base is reflected in the current lack of consensus regarding autonomy of decision making. A staff nurse will often be unable to identify a single decision that is hers and hers alone to make; and if she does, her colleague working by her side cannot be expected to agree. In fact, the only area of agreement regarding nursing's autonomy that this author has consistently found in talking with other nurses is that there is no such thing.

It is no wonder then that the other health professionals involved in the care of the patient are also unable to articulate a single area of decision making that belongs to nurses. Thus, many physicians feel it is their right and duty to write orders governing all aspects of a patient's care, including routine comfort measures, such as 'turn patient every two hours', 'back rub at HS (hour of sleep – bedtime)' and 'routine oral hygiene in am and at HS'.

Peer review of practice and identification with a professional organisation were effectively in place in the United States in the 1920s through the Boards of Registry and Alumnae Associations. Most cities and towns had a Board of Registry comprised of registered nurses. One of the main functions of the board was the assignment of cases to nurses. Physicians or patients needing a private duty nurse called the board, which acted as a clearinghouse for matching up cases with nurses. To be registered with the board for private duty, a nurse had to be a member in good standing of her school's Alumnae Association. This was not always easy to maintain since involvement in almost any kind of scandal (especially if a newspaper mentioned the nurse's name) would often result in the nurse's name being 'stricken from the roles of the graduates'. An example, taken from the actual student records of the Connecticut Training School from the end of the last century, tells of a Miss Happy Jane Daniels, who entered the school in 1884 and was graduated in 1886. The footnote on her student record page read as follows:

> In the autumn of 1888 her name was mentioned in the newspapers in the connection of a divorce of Dr A _____ from his wife. Her name is no longer on our list of graduates. She is married to Dr A _____ and lives in New Haven.

Another function of the board was to receive complaints about a nurse's performance for investigation and action, if any was warranted. Since supervision of a nurse's work after graduation was almost nonexistent, the board functioned similarly to the way local medical societies do today in the performance of 'peer review' of practice.

Finally, the board acted as a standard setter whenever situations occurred for which no precedent had ever been set. Since home care was individualised and unpredictable, it was not uncommon for the board to act as arbiter in cases where a dispute about the efficacy of a nurse's action existed.

Peer review of practice in the 1970s is a foreign concept to most nurses. Because of the hierarchical and authoritarian nature of the bureaucracy, evaluation of performance usually flows from superior to inferior rather than from peer to peer. Staff nurses look to their head nurse to tell them how well or how poorly they are doing. Head nurses look to their supervisors and supervisors to their director of nurses. This author clearly remembers, however, that as a staff nurse, I had a very clear idea of which of my colleagues were good nurses and which ones were not. I was better able to evaluate staff nurses when I was one than later when I was head nurse. The evaluation mechanism in place now, however, assumes that people in superior positions have superior knowledge.

Performance evaluations are supposed to reward excellence and maintain a competent staff by weeding out unsafe and incompetent practitioners. Perhaps if the system functioned more effectively, society would not be clamouring so loudly for better accountability mechanisms. However, in response to society's demands for better acountability, quality assurance programmes are now being designed which use staff nurses for both setting standards and for evaluating staff nurse performance. Establishment of peer review of practice through staff nurse dominated quality assurance programmes will effectively increase the professionalism of nursing practice.

Nursing today suffers from the absence of a single unifying force that has the power to influence significantly the direction in which the health care delivery system moves. Although the American Nurses Association has an every increasing impact on legislation, it often lacks support from nurses (both in terms of individual membership and their active personal support) for the positions it takes on various issues. For a multitude of reasons, nurses today often look to their employing institutions or individuals for leadership on issues affecting role development, health care delivery, standards of nursing practice, and even guidance on moral and ethical issues in which they are involved daily. When nurses were in private duty, the Board of Registry and the Alumnae Association were professional organisations of great significance and power in the life of the nurse. Since nurses became employees of major institutions, no professional organisation has had much impact on the life of the individual nurse.

A comparison of the transition from student to graduate in the 1920s and the same process as we enter the 1980s clearly depicts the effect of both the shift in setting of education and of practice.

Students in the 1920s experienced a training programme similar to the one developed 50 years earlier by Florence Nightingale. The Nightingale school emphasised a two-pronged approach to nursing education: 1) the development of exemplary technical skills in treatment measures and facilitating physical comfort and, 2) the development of personal character of impeccable moral purity. Nightingale believed in strict adherence to the rules and regulations promulgated by school authorities to achieve the desired ends. 'Deviant' behaviour was punished. The emphasis on the development of a 'pure' moral character and the use of step-by-step procedures to teach technical skills may have been appropriate to prepare the original nurse pioneers in the 1860s, but it did little to prepare the modern woman of the 1920s for the variety of situations she faced as an employed private duty nurse.

All aspects of a student nurse's life were subject to scrutiny and control. On duty, she was expected to carry out all orders from her superiors (both nurses and physicians) with absolute accuracy, military precision, and unquestioning obedience. Off duty, she was expected to lead a life of moral purity; no breath of scandal was permitted to mar the unimpeachable character of a nurse. The superintendent of nurses was concerned with how a student nurse looked, who she spoke to, what she said, how she said it, what she read, what she didn't read, what form of recreation she enjoyed (and with whom), what she ate, and how well she slept. Behaviour which did not measure up to the standard was met with swift punishment in the form of either a reprimand or dismissal.

The following comments are excerpted from actual student records and reflect typical responses to student performance that deviated from the established procedures. The importance of an attitude of obedience is obvious.

> While assisting the night nurse in 2 east showed a disposition to do as she thought best—not as she was taught . . . tested temperature of enemata with her hand . . . poured solution by sight, not by measure and in other ways was untrustworthy. Reproved but continued as above, dismissed in consequence.
>
> . . . was severely reprimanded for impertinence to her head nurse . . . and for insubordination when told if she does any more careless work or is impertinent to any one or argues with patients or criticizes those in authority she will be dismissed. Left.
>
> . . . seems in a dream and mind far away . . . has again been reported as very careless in pouring medicines . . . recorded medicines and treatments before they had been given, including treatment for a patient out on pass. When corrected seems to think that 'everyone makes mistakes' . . . careless, heedless methods. Dismissed.
>
> . . . was severely reprimanded . . . she failed to compare a patient's clothing with the list and consequently sent another patient's clothes in the place of the right ones . . . left the treatment room in an unsatisfactory condition and the package of clothing was pinned together instead of tied. These careless methods if repeated would call for even more severe reprimand.
>
> . . . left the medicine cabinet standing open, breaking an important rule. Her excuse was she thought another nurse was going to give medicines was not considered sufficient as serious consequences might have followed. She was called to the office and severely reprimanded.
>
> . . . she is inclined to do things her own way instead of the way she was taught . . . talks a good deal while about her work . . . asks questions at inconvenient times . . . is fond of doing things her own way, but has improved in her manner of taking reproach . . . failed to carry out orders . . . was severely reproved and told that the offense would be entered in the records against her . . . has not improved but rather gone backward . . . the head nurse dares not leave her in the ward without supervision . . . she was found very unsatisfactory and dropped.[1]

While failing to conform to established procedures was considered a grievous offence, nothing was more serious than conduct viewed as unbecoming a professional nurse. Consider the following examples:

> The past three months has not done well . . . she had been noisy, boisterous, talking in a loud tone of voice. She was reproved for this but in a few weeks other reports were brought to me. She made trouble among the nurses by telling stories and gossiping about them . . . her conduct on the street and in the Hospital was unprofessional . . . she went to one of the restaurants with a medical student where liquor was sold but claimed she did not drink any. Dismissed.

> . . . was reprimanded for lingering in the corridor when off duty in the evening. She acknowledged that she was talking with one of the house doctors. Though warned of the consequences, went out one evening with a house doctor, till 1:30 a.m., tried to enter the dormitory through a window. She was called before a special committee and as there could be no extenuation of her conduct, she was expelled from the school.

> Dismissed, not up to our standard . . . would call out of her window to passersby . . . very familiar with young men about the hospital . . . undesirable in every way.

> Was seen sitting on the floor by the surgical carriage laughing and talking with a patient and another nurse. She was reprimanded for such frivolity and taken from the ward. She violated the most ordinary sense of propriety.

This education did little to prepare a young woman for the challenges and uncertainties she faced as a graduate nurse in private practice. First, there was the uncertainty of the future. If she was on a case, it might last for one day, one week, one month, one year, or longer. However long the duration, the nurse was expected to be on duty all day, every day. A day off could be enjoyed only after a suitable replacement had been secured. When not on a case, the nurse had no assurance whatsoever of whether the next call would come in one day, one week, one month, or never. Thus, from a student life of virtually complete minute-by-minute regulation, the graduate went to a life which alternated between total unpredictability and unremitting constancy. The financial insecurity of this employment situation is obvious.

Another area of uncertainty was the type of equipment and supplies available in the home for use in the care of the patient. The rigid adherence to regulations in the performance of procedures as a student did little to prepare the graduate nurse for the level of innovativeness and adaptability demanded of her in private practice. Some nurses owned a few of the more basic pieces of equipment, but in general the application of comfort measures and treatment procedures required the ability to use everyday household items as sick-room equipment.

The presence or absence of electricity, running water, toilets, bathing facilities, cooking ranges, ice boxes, etc., were factors that significantly affected her practice. The establishment of routine procedures carried over from one household to another was virtually impossible, since, for one thing, electricity and plumbing were just becoming standard household features. Although nothing in her training prepared the nurse to be either flexible or adaptable, the circumstances of care were so variable that case-to-case similarities could not be much relied on.

Finally, the nurse faced untold uncertainties surrounding her ability to establish therapeutic relationships. Nothing in her education prepared her to understand the wide ranges of behaviours that exists in the real world. The narrowness of her education, particularly the Victorian interpretation of morality, scarcely provided her with a context for understanding human nature. Thus, the ultimate uncertainty she faced was whether or not she would be able to establish and maintain a relationship with the patient and family that would enable her to affect the outcomes of the illness successfully.

Thus, the transition from student nurse to graduate nurse in the 1920s was necessarily one of role expansion. Nursing was learned in a setting that was rigid, militaristic, and religiously oriented in an institution governed by rules and regulations dictating all facets of one's work and one's personal life. Nursing was practised in a setting where differences, variations, unpredictability and uncertainty were the norm and where creativity, adaptability, flexibility and ingenuity were absolute requirements for a successful practice. The system certainly did not guarantee the education of good nurses but, by its very weaknesses, it ensured the 'survival of the fittest'.

The transition from student nurse to graduate nurse in the 1970s was one of role deprivation. Consider the contrast. Education now takes place in institutions of higher education where academic freedom instead of the authority of the superintendent governs curriculum content. Well-prepared faculty design courses to meet objectives which are consistent with the philosophy and theoretical framework of the school. The faculty has a great deal of freedom to choose the appropriate techniques to achieve the educational goals. Students quickly become aware of the level of professional development the faculty has achieved. This awareness initiates the socialisation process of the student as a professional using the faculty as a role model. Unfortunately, the role modelled is one of professional educator rather than professional nurse, but neither students nor faculty are aware of the importance of the difference. It is one thing to be a successful professional educator in an institution of higher education; it is quite something else to be a successful professional nurse, as a staff nurse in an acute care hospital.

Nursing is no longer taught using a step-by-step procedure approach; as a matter of fact, many schools teach virtually no procedures as such, but rather a process of nursing. Upon graduation, the student enters the health system as staff nurse in an institution that is rule and regulation dominated, where deviations from policy are punishable offences, and where the word 'nursing process' is met by an icy stare. Task accomplishment has high priority in hospital nursing.

Since nursing is now taught in institutions whose primary purpose is teaching 'why' rather than 'how', the scope of learning is much broader. Liberal arts courses comprise a major component of every generic baccalaureate programme; hospital schools and associate degree programmes have similarly broadened their scope. Today's students spend short periods of time on the floors, but are exposed to a wide variety of experiences and learning opportunities. They are exposed to a breadth of knowledge unheard of seventy years ago, but to relatively few of the technical skills considered essential in the 1920s. In fact, clinical judgment skills, complex techniques, and in some cases, routine comfort measures are considered appropriate 'first job' learning experiences. The art and skill of hands-on nursing has thus become an on-the-job learning experience, with economic and sociological ramifications for the profession which have weakened rather than broadened it.

Students are taught to provide comprehensive patient care based on a process of nursing using problem-solving skills to develop an individualised plan of care. The case method of patient assignment is used and a student typically cares for one or two patients on any given day. Patients are selected on the basis of a student's learning needs, as perceived by the clinical instructor.

Throughout the education programme, freedom of thought and intellectual curiosity are encouraged; kudos is given to students who challenge policies that restrict individualisation of care. The bright, inquisitive, aggressive student who challenges established procedures with the innocence of ignorance is cherished by her teachers and rewarded for being courageous and willing to question the establishment. Some see these seekers of truth as the vanguard of a revolutionary force for change that will march forward on graduation days for years to come, prepared to modify the health care delivery system for the good of nursing, and, thus, ultimately for the good of the patient care. (If nurses are happy, patient care is bound to be better!)

With the unbounded altruism that typically leads a person into nursing in the first place thus enflamed by the fires of idealism, the new graduate applies for her first staff nurse job in an acute care hospital. As a staff nurse, she finds herself in a position of powerlessness. The job description for her position describes little of what she really does; she may find, however, it can be used to add tasks indiscriminately to her workload. The position of staff nurse is viewed by other professionals in the hospital as the lowest in the pecking order of power. Unfortunately, this attitude is also prevalent in the hierarchy of the many nursing departments where, despite all protestation to the contrary, the attitude of 'she's just a staff nurse' is still all too common. Our would-be revolutionary, so recently armed with the weapons of change, finds herself in one of the most powerless positions in the hospital. Her superiors do not expect her to be a change agent; perish the thought. If she can learn what she has to know to do the job, especially how to not 'rock the boat', her chances of success and promotion are secure. The speed with which she learns her place will affect how soon she will be rewarded for being a 'good nurse'.

The modern hospital can still be described in the same language used to describe hospitals in the 1920s: militaristic, authoritarian, bureaucratic institutions governed by rules and regulations, called policies and procedures, administered in a structure of authoritarianism that borders on the absolute. The aspiring professional nurse finds herself powerless in a power-dominated system where power rests in the highest positions and only those closest to the seats of power are highly valued. Unfortunately, nothing in her education, including the faculty's professional role modelling, prepared the new nurse to cope successfully with the reality of this powerlessness, let alone to affect change in the face of it.

The problem of role deprivation so aptly described by Marlene Kramer[2] is one of the most devastating problems nursing faced as it came into the 1980s. Thirty per cent of the best educated practitioners in nursing changed careers within two years of graduation. Our profession was in serious trouble.

The transition from student to graduate in the 1920s and in the 1970s accurately reflects how the change of practice setting led to the deprofessionalisation of nursing. In the 1920s, the transition was out of necessity an expansion from a skill-based, narrow education to an independent practice containing many of the characteristics of a profession. By the 1970s we find the situation reversed. Broad based, professionally oriented programmes produce nurses who then go on to fill impotent roles, constricted within rigid sets of rules and regulations. This can be attributed primarily to the change in the setting of practice to the hospital, with its predictably bureaucratic power structure. To regain the element of professionalism nursing once had it is necessary to create a *delivery* system that lives up to the expectations created by contemporary education and facilitates professional practice. That system is Primary Nursing.

THE 1920s, 1930s, 1940s, 1950s AND 1960s

What has happened to nursing since the 1920s that paints such a bleak picture? An oversupply of nurses resulted in underemployment in the 1920s and yet by the 1950s and 1960s there were severe shortages, reflecting profound changes in society. From a private practice conducted in patient's homes nursing made the tremendous leap into an enormously complex machine and space age health care practice conducted in one of the most complicated institutions known to mankind. To answer the 'what happened?' question, we need to look at nursing's reaction to the world events that shaped the course of practice.

THE 1920s

In the wake of the First World War, women moved one step closer to liberation by getting the right to vote. The idea of a career appealed to more and more of them, and nursing was viewed as a highly acceptable alternative to teaching. It was just as respectable as a career and still a cut above the other types of employment then available to young women who did not wish to teach. There was no shortage of educational opportunities and the cost was within the means of most middle-class families.

New schools of nursing were springing up everywhere, as newly constructed hospitals, many of them small, private organisations which appreciated the economic advantages of student labour, initiated their own training centres. In 1926, there were 2,155 schools of nursing in the United States compared to 1,300 in 1946.[3]

THE 1930s

The nurse-power over-supply had kept salaries down, so nurses were poorly prepared to endure the economic hardships of the depression of 1929. Scarce jobs became scarcer as fewer families could afford to feed themselves, let alone hire nurses to care for their sick. The use of hospitals for the care of the ill increased. By the early 1930s, nurses were standing in the bread lines and eating in soup kitchens, unable to find enough work to support themselves. During this period, many of them returned to their home hospitals and asked to be allowed to work in exchange for room and board. The hospitals opened their doors to their own graduates and, in exchange for a full week of work, gave them a place to sleep and three meals a day. Although graduate nurses had worked in hospitals prior to this period it was in the capacity of private duty nurses, not as employees of the hospital. As time passed, these nurses were paid a stipend and their role was eventually legitimised by the establishment of job descriptions and regular salaries. At first, however, there was an interesting confusion over the difference there should be in the job description between a senior nursing student and a graduate nurse. After all, talented seniors were head nurses of the wards and in some hospitals even took over when the superintendent of nurses had a day off. Not surprisingly there was concern over the use of salaried graduate nurses in positions which could equally be filled by cheaper student labour. It was under these circumstances that the shift in setting of graduate practice from home to hospital now took place. Never since has the majority of trained practitioners been in private practice.

Since graduate nurses could technically perform all the care a patient required, the case method was used for patient assignments. Individualised patient care was still the focus of their attention; the difference between home care and hospital care was negligible. However, this did mark the first time that graduate nurse practice was subject to the rules and regulations that exist in a bureaucratic institution.

THE 1940s

Before the nation recovered economically from the effects of the depression, Pearl Harbor was bombed.

The wartime need for trained nurses quickly assumed a priority second only to the need for armed servicemen. Periodically throughout the war serious consideration was given to drafting nurses; the problem, however, was an inadequate supply of trained nurses rather than an unwillingness of those trained to serve. Overnight the oversupply turned into a critical shortage. The federal government heavily subsidised nursing education and the Cadet Corps training programmes began producing nurses in unprecedented numbers.

Still, no matter how many were trained, the war required more and more. To relieve the continuing shortage multi-level training programmes were developed to teach auxiliary personnel how to perform simple care and technical procedures. In the military services, these programmes produced 'corpsmen' specially trained for each branch of the armed services at various levels of technical skill. In civilian life two types of auxiliary training programmes were developed: a one-year programme preparing people to provide technical nursing care, and on-the-job training which prepared people to perform the simplest types of care. The former were called licensed practical nurses, the latter, nurses' aides. Nurses' aide training programmes were originally designed and taught by the American Red Cross for housewives who volunteered their time to relieve the extreme nurse shortage in civilian hospitals. These original volunteer aides were often identified by the colour of their smocks and so became known as the 'grey ladies' or the 'pink ladies'. By the end of World War II, this role had been institutionalised to the extent that most hospitals were providing their own on-the-job training programmes for nurse aides. Indeed, for a while, some hospitals had two aide job descriptions: one for paid aides and one for unpaid, or volunteer aides. Simultaneously the licensed practical nurses found a permanent place in the hospital hierarchy.

Meanwhile, wartime acquisition of medical knowledge and technological developments grew tremendously, resulting in enormous increases in the size and complexity of hospitals. New developments and techniques acquired on the battlefield were brought back to the home front as quickly as the knowledge could be acquired and the nature of care given in hospitals changed beyond recognition, especially in the fragmentation of complex procedures.

Towards the end of the war, as projections were being made for peacetime needs, nursing leaders feared that nursing would once again suffer the economic hardships experienced before the war. The phenomenal number of cadet nurses returning to the United States, coupled with the unprecedented preparation of auxiliary workers trained in many of the simpler aspects of hospital care, was expected to drive salaries down to pre-war levels. In the event, of course, this did not happen. Instead, the overwhelming shortage of nurses persisted and was a major concern to providers of health care for the next 20 years.

THE 1950s

Much of the nursing research of the 1950s was devoted to developing delivery systems for acute care settings that would facilitate the use of auxiliary workers (LPNs and NAs) in providing direct nursing care under the supervision of registered nurses. In 1948, Esther Lucille Brown[4] exhorted the profession to develop ways to use the people already trained and pleaded for the establishment of nursing services that were differentiated but integrated. The resulting development projects and research efforts culminated in the design of team nursing.

The post-war building boom experienced throughout the country was especially great in the hospital industry. To make sure that adequate beds were available the federal government passed the Hill-Burton Act to furnish new buildings. Hospitals were erected in communities that had previously had none and wings were added to existing buildings. During these years, health manpower education and training programmes could not begin to keep up with the increase in hospital beds. Ever greater pressures were exerted on the nursing profession to prepare more and more registered nurses. Many hospitals had whole wings or floors that were unoccupied because of insufficient staff.

Throughout the United States and Canada, the late 1950s and the 1960s were years of trouble and frustration for staff nurses and nurse administrators. The post-war shortage of nurses became a chronic problem that threatened to hold back the unprecedented growth in medicine and hospitals. The shortages were of nurses, not dollars. Recruitment competition was fierce. Attractions such as low-cost housing, tuition-free courses, and free holiday weekends became standard incentives. One hospital located in the heart of 'automobile city' offered graduates options on cars bearing the same name as the hospital. The recruitment ads in journals looked like marriage broker ads.

The problem of the chronic under-supply of nurses coupled with the unprecedented growth in hospital beds was compounded by: 1) the ever increasing complexity of new technological procedures and 2) a persistently high turnover of nurses.

> A recent study of some 325 hospitals showed that about 20 percent of the positions for professional nurses were vacant, as were 18 percent of the positions for practical nurses. In New York City, over half of the positions for professional nurses in the public hospitals were unfilled in 1961. In all hospitals in Los Angeles, private as well as public, 25 to 30 percent of the positions for professional staff nurses are reported as unfilled. In a recent survey of all general hospitals in the State of Massachusetts, it was found that 20 percent of the positions for professional staff nurses were not filled.[5]

These vacancies were in existing financed positions, not wishful dreams! The modern nurses of the 1950s had become mobile. It seemed as though suddenly they had discovered that they could move to any corner of the US and find a nursing job. The shortage was nation-wide. A nurse employed in a hospital with short staffing could resign, move to another part of the country, and count on being employed by another hospital with an equally severe problem; only the scenery was different. The number of nurses who did just this caused a turnover rate that created appalling staffing problems for nurse managers. These chronic shortages and high turnover rates among nurses led in turn to an increased reliance on the more stable caregivers in nursing's workforce: aides, orderlies and licensed practical nurses.

> This pragmatic solution to the problem of shortages has produced an alarming dilution of the quality of services. In some hospitals the use of auxiliary workers has reached such extreme proportions that nursing aides give as much as 80% of the direct nursing services.[6]

The need to utilise these auxiliary workers was undeniable; the challenge to nursing was to create an organisation for them at the station level that would facilitate their maximal utilisation under the control and supervision of registered nurses.

During the 1950s, the concept of team nursing in its present sense developed and swept the country. By the mid-1960s, if a hospital was not using this model, its nursing care was considered inferior by the nursing community. In implementing team nursing, hospitals divided stations of any size into two teams, each to be directed by a registered nurse called a 'team leader', on two, if not all three, shifts. The team leader supervised and coordinated all the nursing care activities performed by team members who were usually LPNs, and nurses' aides, and sometimes RNs. For example, the team leader was responsible for seeing to it that everything ordered for all the patients on her team was administered in a timely fashion. In addition to these 'foreman' activities, the team leader was responsible for providing professional direction in the care rendered by the less prepared team members.

To nurse administrators obsessed with the problems of nurse shortages this seemed an ideal way to utilise RNs maximally; to hospital administrators, team nursing appeared a way to hold down professional salary costs by using cheaper labour, and, to at least some nurses, it created a role that enabled them to be one step removed from what was perceived as the menial work of bedside nursing. *Most* nurses really lamented being removed from bedside care, but to be against team nursing in the 1960s was like being opposed to moon walks in the 1970s.

THE 1960s

By the mid-1960s, the roar of dissatisfaction had reach a crescendo. Patients were dissatisfied with hospital care, physicians were dissatisfied with nursing, and nurses were dissatisfied with themselves and everyone else. The public used the popular press as a forum to express its unhappiness with hospital care. Nurses expressed theirs by continuing to switch hospitals, by leaving hospital nursing, and by leaving nursing altogether with alarming frequency. In large hospitals, it was not unheard of to run 500 nurses through orientation programmes in one year! During the mid-1960s this author studied some characteristics of the nursing staff at the University of Minnesota Hospitals and found the average length of time a new graduate stayed on the job was seven months. In some positions there was a 300 per cent turnover—three nurses in one position in one year. Kramer's work accurately describes the dimensions of the problem.[7]

Nurse administrators faced two major problems: 1) patients were receiving fragmented, depersonalised and discontinuous care, and 2) nurses were discouraged and frustrated with their jobs. Unfortunately, the two problems were, and often still are, treated as one. The belief seems to be that if the profession of nursing is strong and healthy (and nurses are happy) then patients will naturally receive better nursing care. This may or may not be true. The juxtaposition of the two problems leads to a concentration of all energy and attention on solving nurses' problems, and not enough on the problems of poor patient care.

Within nursing the focus was now on the concept of professionalism. Efforts to define the word 'professional' came to centre on a differentiation based on the educational preparation of practitioners. Two-year community college-based schools of nursing began replacing the hospital diploma programmes, enabling a clearer delineation of levels of preparation. The American Nurses Association position paper of 1965 used the word 'professional' to describe the practice of nurses who had been graduated from baccalaureate programmes and 'technical' to describe the practice of a graduate of an associate degree or diploma programme.[8] An unfortunate result of the position paper has been the obscuring of the basic meaning of the word 'professional'.

Meanwhile, efforts were being made to isolate the 'unique' body of knowledge that would 'belong' to nursing and to nursing only. Frequent curriculum revisions became the rule rather than the exception and as the clinical component of nursing was de-emphasised, confusion and ambiguity concerning its boundaries inevitably grew. Nurse educators and administrators disagreed widely about the appropriate content of nurse education programmes. Today the divergence in expectations of new graduates between educators and administrators is so wide many fear the chasm that exists can never be bridged.

At the graduate level nursing education swung, within a period of a very few years, from functional (education or administration) to clinical (medical/surgical, maternal-child, pediatric, and psychiatric nursing, etc.). Clinical specialists prepared at the master's level arrived in hospitals and nurse administrators began the still unfinished search for an appropriate job description that would ensure the most effective utilisation of this most highly educated clinical nurse.

Because the problems within nursing and the problem in taking care of hospitalised sick people were often seen as one and the same, the ferment in nursing education had a powerful effect on nursing service. Some nurse administrators, in an attempt to implement the position paper of the American Nurses Association, tried to reserve the team leader role for graduate nurses with 'BSN' after their names. The 'professional nurse' was seen as the RN with a baccalaureate education who was prepared to develop a comprehensive care plan 'based on nursing process' (sic). The morale problems created when someone without a bachelor's degree was hired as a team leader were very depressing. The efforts to define professional practice on the basis of educational credentials in the 1960s left a legacy of second-class citizenship issues in the 1970s that promise to remain with us for many decades to come.

Nurse administrators, mindful of the efforts to identify the unique body of knowledge that is nursing's alone, and in an effort to solve the staff shortage problem, began to analyse the non-nursing activities being undertaken by nurses. Activities that were clearly non-nursing tasks were freely given away to other departments. So, in the 1960s, nurses stopped washing beds of discharged patients, and housekeeping departments began cleaning all kinds of substances, even material produced by the human body. Pharmacy departments began automatic replacement programmes for floor stocks of medications, dietary departments began passing nourishment and drinking water, and laboratory services began doing venipunctures. New tasks were no longer delegated to nurses just because physicians were no longer interested in performing them. Requests for nurses to accept delegated medical tasks were now subject to new scrutiny by nursing administration and if certain criteria were not met, the tasks did not become nursing responsibilities. If a delegated medical task (DMT) did not seem to 'belong' to the 'unique' field of nursing, responsibility for its performance was not accepted by the nursing department. (However, by the time a director of nursing received the request to train floor nurses to perform a new task, such as taking central venous pressures, she usually discovered, to her chagrin, that intensive care unit (ICU) nurses had been doing it for Dr So-and-so for the past six months.) Since there was no consensus about the content of the unique field of nursing, the decision about whether or not to take on a new DMT was usually decided in the negative because of workload impact. When the starting of intravenous drips (IVs) was no longer an intern's job, special IV teams were developed because nursing could not take on that additional workload. As intermittent positive pressure treatments became popular, new departments of inhalation/respiratory therapy developed. Indeed, many hospitals went so far as to train lay people to administer medications to patients in an effort to relieve the workload of the registered nurses. The transference of 'non-nursing' tasks to other departments, and the development of special teams to perform therapies too time-consuming for floor nurses were some of the means used to offset the excessive demands being placed on the inadequate supply of nursing resources. The establishment of unit management departments to relieve nurses of paperwork was another avenue vigorously pursued by hospital and nursing administrators in the latter half of the 1960s to 'free the nurse to nurse'.

Nurses thus 'freed', however, were still so harried and harassed trying to cope with the army of caregivers that arrived on the station each day, that patients were frequently heard apologising before they requested an essential service from the rushed nurses: 'I know you're busy but. . .' The coordination of the army was difficult since nurses had no real authority over them; however, when something went wrong it was easy to know whom to blame since the nurse was the one with the cap on. (Significantly by 1968 staff nurses and nurse administrators in many hospitals were locked in battle over the issue of whether or not the wearing of caps was mandatory.)

By the late 1960s, the majority of clinical bedside care was being given by NAs and LPNs, supervised by RNs who also performed some of the more complex tasks, such as adding medications to the IVs. Hordes of technicians requiring information and coordination arrived daily on the station at their department's convenience to perform technical procedures on patients. As caps and uniforms ceased to identify who was performing which services and functions, patients became thoroughly confused about who was doing what for them. Although nurses were spending more and more time in communication-related activities it became less and less realistic to expect a team leader to know the names and diagnoses of the patients on her team! It is not unfair to say that patients did not know which caregivers were nurses, and nurses did not know who their patients were or why they were in the hospital.

SOLUTIONS OF THE 1960s

Two of the most popular solutions put forth during the 1960s were unit management, in which non-nurses managed many stations, and more nurses. Since patients' loudest complaints were about dehumanised care, and nurses' loudest complaints were about insufficient help and too much paperwork, nurse administrators concentrated on getting more nurses and reducing the clerical chores. The assumption was that this would result in better patient care, or happy nurses equal happy patients! By 1967, the University of Minnesota Hospitals were ready to give serious consideration to developing a department of unit management. This author and other nurses visited hospitals in various states to study their experiences before launching such a department ourselves.

Accompanying us on these trips was an associate hospital administrator. At each hospital he would ask his counterpart two questions: 'How much does unit management cost in new salary dollars?' and 'What effect has it had on patient care?' We were dismayed when the answer to the first question was, in some cases, as much as $500,000 in new salaries with no commensurate reduction in the nursing budget. But the answer to the second question was even more discouraging. The few hospitals that had conducted before-and-after studies of how nursing time was utilised found that there was little or no significant change in the amount of time devoted to direct patient care. I had great difficulty understanding and accepting this fact. In hospitals where virtually all the paperwork was handled by non-nurses, not to mention such functions as supply-ordering, equipment and environmental maintenance, nurses were still not spending more time with patients; I began to wonder if it was a matter of being *able* or being *willing*.

As I began analysing this question I searched the literature to develop a better understanding of the relationship between staffing and the quality of care. An Investigation of the Relation between Nursing Activity and Patient Welfare, a study done by Myrtle Kitchell Aydelotte at the University of Iowa, produced some startling results.[9] Staffing was varied repeatedly by changing ratios of RNs to LPNs to nurses' aides and numbers of station personnel. Data were collected before and after each staffing change to determine what effect different patterns had on the quantity and quality of the care the patients received. The most startling finding (consistent with the others, but more dramatic) was the design whereby professional staff assigned to a patient care unit was increased by sixty per cent. Measurements of the amount of time the greatly expanded staff spent with patients were made and *there was no significant increase*! The sixty per cent more time available was spent on the station, but *not in the patients' rooms*! It was spent at the desk, in the lavatory, at coffee, charting, talking to house staff, etc. Anywhere, but *not in the patients' rooms!*

Thus, it seemed that neither of the two popular solutions to the problems of hospital nursing services was really effective; neither unit management nor more nurses necessarily had the desired effect of increasing the amount of time nurses spent caring for patients or of ensuring greater patient satisfaction with that care. The solutions did create more time but it was not spent at the bedside.

And so the question became: Was the nurse shortage one of actual numbers of nurses or was it a problem in the ways nurses were being utilised? Once that question began receiving serious attention, energy formerly directed at recruitment, turnover, scheduling, etc., began being applied to an analysis of what nurses actually did and how they did it.

At the University of Minnesota, staff nurses and leaders working on the unit management project station (by now called 'Project 32', so named because the pilot station was number 32), focused attention on that question and decided that before any major modification in hospital structure, such as a unit management department, was undertaken, efforts should be made to streamline the delivery of nursing service. The intent was to ensure appropriate utilisation of nurses under unit management while avoiding the expensive pitfalls in the systems used by other hospitals.

It should be noted that this attention was still focused on ways to improve the implementation of *team* nursing. There was a strong feeling that more effective team nursing (following the book's directions more exactly) would certainly result in better planned, more coordinated and more comprehensive patient care.

In an effort to discover just how team nursing had been incorrectly implemented, three major problem areas were identified and concentrated upon: 1) the fragmentation of care; 2) complex channels of communication; and 3) shared responsibility and lack of accountability. Efforts to solve these problems by improving the implementation of team nursing were as unsuccessful in this instance as they had been in all others. However, in this case they led to the establishment of an alternative organisation which eventually came to be called Primary Nursing. Its design was a direct reaction to the inability of the team system to deliver nursing care that was coordinated, individualised, and comprehensive; instead of fragmented care, the case method is used; instead of complex channels of communication, simple direct patterns are used; instead of shared responsibility, individual responsibility is clearly allocated.

PROBLEMS OF TEAM NURSING

Fragmentation of care

Team nursing was supposed to facilitate effective utilisation of auxiliary workers (LPNs and NAs) under the direct supervision of registered nurses. To accomplish this tasks were *divided up into the simplest components*, and then graded and matched to the skill levels of these workers. Thus, nurses' aides took all the temperatures; LPNs took all the blood pressures; registered nurses passed all the medications. From the patient's point of view, this form of work allocation required relating to at least three and usually many more members of the staff on each of the three daily shifts. When work assignments are divided in this way the reward and punishment structure that motivates individuals centres primarily on their timely completion. Thus, the aide who is taking the 11 o'clock temperatures is in a hurry to complete them so she can help pass lunch trays that arrive at 11.20. Similarly, the registered nurse passing the 9.00 am medications is in a hurry to get them out on time otherwise 'meds will be late' and the ugly question of whether or not there was an 'error' due to lateness may have to be addressed. Patients requesting personal care of this aide or RN are soon made to realise that their care needs are *interrupting* important work assignments. The underlying assumption here seems to be that if all of the different bits of care are administered on time (which is, in any case, obviously not always possible) patients will have received good, comprehensive care. The fundamental flaws in this assumption demand close scrutiny.

Complex channels of communication

The fragmentation of care that resulted from a task-based method of work assignment led to the second problem of *complex communication channels*. As we examined further what nurses did and how they did it at our hospital, we found inordinate amounts of time being spent in activities related to communication. Despite this, however, I remained uneasy about the amount of knowledge nursing staff members actually had about their patients. As the communication problem was studied, we found highly complex patterns in use in shift reports. The following example depicts the magnitude of the problem:

On one busy surgical station, the head nurse often arrived a half hour early (to get a head start) and received the morning report from the night nurse. She then relayed the report to the team leaders who later gave it to team members. Patient condition information was thus sifted through three minds and subjective evaluations before it became data to be used by those giving direct care to the patients. At the end of the shift, the process was reversed; team members would tell their team leader what had been going on all day with their patients, the team leader would report to the head nurse who would report to the evening charge nurse who would report to the evening team leaders who would eventually give the patient condition report to the evening team members.

Another example of the complexity of the communication channels was seen in an examination of the typical reactions to a change in the patient's condition. The team member who observed the condition change in the patient reported it to the team leader (who might or might not verify it personally). The team leader would then tell the head nurse, who called the physician; he would tell the head nurse what actions to take, which she would pass on to the team leader who would then tell the team member taking care of the patient what to do about it. In identifying this elaborate hierarchy of information channels in team nursing it was obvious to many of us that despite all of these time-consuming reporting and communication mechanisms, the people actually administering the care did so *with little or no knowledge either of the patient or the problem* for which he was being treated. As one Primary Nurse said:

> I did team nursing before where one person took the vitals, another person passed the meds and you really didn't get to know your patients and what was going on with them and you were lucky if at the end of the day you had enough information to pass on to the next shift and you really didn't have the full and complete picture but just bits and pieces of it.

Shared responsibility and lack of accountability

The third difficulty which we identified and tried to correct in team nursing was eventually seen as having three interrelated aspects: 1) the problem of *shared responsibility*; 2) the problem of *the blank space under the words 'nursing care plan'*; and 3) the problem of *the role of the team leader*.

The problem of shared responsibility can be looked at both as it applied to completing the tasks of care and as it applied to care plans. The team leader assigned all the tasks, but she was also responsible for making sure that everything was done on time. So, if a team member forgot to perform a certain procedure when it was due, she could always say to the team leader, 'You forgot to remind me'. This sharing of responsibility for performing care tasks meant that if something was not done, no one person could be blamed. Shared responsibility equals no responsibility.

Care plans have always created problems, but especially so in team nursing. In the first place, a care plan is supposed to be the result of a care conference. Everybody on the team is supposed to contribute to its development. (The clear implication was that no one member of the team was smart enough to develop a plan by herself.) Since there are only five days a week when conferences can be scheduled, five care plans would be the most that could be generated. This, coupled with a high turnover of patients, always made it impossible to achieve the dream of an up-to-date care plan for each patient. But no team leader need feel too bad about not having a full complement of care plans because when she went off duty, another nurse with the same imprecise degree of responsibility assumed the same role with the same limitations. Everybody was responsible for all patients, so no one was responsible for any one patient.

The blank space under the words 'nursing care plan' is a problem that has consumed the time, attention and energy of large segments of nursing's leadership

2765

for the past 30 years. They might well have asked who dreamed up the idea in the first place because it certainly does not derive from a need consciously identified by staff nurses.

No other single issue, thought, technique, problem, or phenomenon in nursing has received as much attention, has been as much written about, taught, talked about, worked at, read about and cried over, with so little success. No other issue in nursing has caused so much guilt-energy to be misspent. Yet, no other piece of paper in a hospital system is as devoid of information as that entitled 'nursing care plan' unless Joint Commission* is coming or students have recently worked on the floor.

Why? How do new graduates learn to give adequate care so quickly without using the basic tool upon which their educational process was based? Anyone who has spent any amount of time in nursing service at any level in any reasonably good hospital knows that, in fact, top-drawer nursing care can be delivered without nursing care plans. Nursing care plans present one of the most stubborn problems faced by modern nursing and it seems that no matter what is said, done or written about them, their use still remains a serious problem. Why has it been so intractable?

First of all, I do not believe nurses avoid writing care plans because they do not care about the continuity of nursing care, nor do I believe that lack of time is the real reason for the blankness of that piece of paper. Anyone who has been in nursing service for any length of time knows that there are many reasons and many excuses given as to why the plans are not consistently completed. Among the most popular of these are:

Not enough staff.
They take too long.
Nobody reads them.
They get outdated too soon.
Nursing care plans are not a part of the permanent record and, therefore, not important.
Nursing care plans are a part of the permanent record and, therefore, of limited value as a communication tool.
The head nurse doesn't pay any attention to them, so why should I bother?
The head nurse doesn't care if they're done or not.
We give good care without them.

Of all these reasons/excuses, inadequate time is the most difficult to refute and,

* This refers to an accrediting group that audits hospital functions and approves (or disapproves) the hospital on the basis of compliance with the standards established by the Commission.

therefore, the one most frequently used. To be sure, nurses never have enough time to give the kind of care they would like to give. However, it is also true that nursing care plans are the easiest responsibility to neglect since the system offers no immediate sanctions for failing to complete them.

With the shared responsibility and lack of accountability inherent in team nursing, everyone can feel guilty about the absence of care plans, as witness the great variety of excuses, but no one really has to do anything about them. One Primary Nurse commented:

> I was finding that in team nursing a lot of things were getting missed and that a lot of people weren't caring about these things getting missed. There were a few people who really cared but they knew it couldn't make a difference when there were so many that didn't care. Here it seems like everybody really cares about their patients. In team nursing they could just pass the buck. Things could just be moving along from one shift to the next but here everyone is really responsible and here everyone is so happy.

The third aspect of the problem of shared responsibility is the role of the team leader. It is most easily illustrated by the challenge a head nurse faces in the orientation of a new graduate. The latter usually has to be taught how to be an effective team leader as quickly as possible so that the staff nurse vacancy which has existed for some time can be filled as quickly as possible. Anxious to practise her newly acquired nursing skills in her first real nursing job, she may or may not have had some experience as a team leader during her student experience. At any rate, the pressure is on both of them to groom her for the role as quickly as possible.

The first thing the new graduate has to learn is how to listen to and retain great masses of verbally transmitted data at morning report. The information may be needed at any time during the coming shift or not at all, but she must still be prepared to retrieve any of it from her brain cells at a moment's notice. The data may be clinical, social, factual and/or impressionistic and be about a large number of patients. Others can forget; the team leader cannot.

Next, our new graduate must be taught how to make out daily assignments. She first must learn the job description limitations that exist for LPNs and aides, and then she must learn the *real* limitations—who can actually do what and how much help various team members will require. In learning who should take care of which patients the new graduate will be taught not to assign herself to any patients if she can possibly avoid it. In this way she will be free to help everyone and make sure that all the work is being accomplished according to schedule. However, if staffing is very low, she learns that she may have to assign herself to a few patients. If so, she is instructed to take those who are least seriously ill so she can be as free as possible to supervise the work of the other team members. Thus, the RN, who is the ranking professional on the team, is steered toward the care of those who need least help.

Next, there is 'rounds with a purpose'. When I left team nursing there were still hot discussions on whether or not rounds could be incorporated with the administration of medication, or if separate rounds 'with a purpose' were not more beneficial. I never really did understand the 'purpose' but I am sure there was one.

The new graduate has to learn how to schedule staggered coffee breaks for the team members and to schedule lunch periods so the staff gets to eat without jeopardising lunch tray deliveries. Afternoon cleaning chores also have to be assigned along with special procedures and new admissions.

Finally, the team leader has to learn how to check with the team members at the end of the shift to find out how all the patients have fared that day, so she can give a comprehensive report to the evening team leader. When the new graduate is able to accomplish all that and get everyone off duty by 3.30 pm (because the hospital surely does not want to pay overtime), then the head nurse can say, 'Wow, she's good!' It is entirely possible that neither she nor, for that matter, the new graduate, has had an opportunity to assess in any meaningful way the quality of clinical judgment our new head nurse brings to the bedside.

It is fair to say that team nursing is a delivery system for nursing that requires enormous amounts of time to be spent in communication, but where it is not expected that nurses will know the diagnosis of a patient. It is a system that takes the individual with the highest licence to care for the sick and tells that person to care for no sick people except the least seriously ill. It is a system in which what is assigned is not patient care, but tasks. The assumption is that if all of these are done on time, especially morning baths, patients are getting good care.

In 1964, during the heyday of team nursing, the author was asked by her director of nursing to study one particular station at a major teaching hospital where the head nurse was having problems managing patient care. The method used to study the station was described in the United States Public Health Service booklet entitled *How to Study Activities in a Patient Unit*.[10] The following excerpts from that report depict typical problems experienced with team nursing.

> Presently, each team member has responsibility for the care of seventeen to eighteen patients. This care is given by three to five team members who have varying levels of skills and education. With a team this large, the activities team leaders have time for are assigning patients to team members, administering medication, doing treatments on patients assigned to nurse aides, charting, giving and receiving verbal communication about patients, and periodically

checking patients' conditions. They do not usually have time to accompany doctors on rounds, to teach patients about pre- or post-operative care, to conduct team conferences, or to acquire an understanding of the psychosocial aspects of the patients' illnesses.

. . . team leaders need an opportunity to acquire information about, and understanding of, the medical care plan. They should be able to accompany doctors on rounds and become familiar with the medical plan. This is essential if nursing care is to be coordinated with the patient's medical treatment . . . the nursing staff is often caring for patients without current information about the medical plan.

This activity analysis showed team leaders spending *less than half their time* with patients while the other half was spent communicating about patient care and handling equipment and supplies.[11]

The first attempt to solve these three problems focused on improvements in the implementation of team nursing, with the goal of providing humane, individualised, comprehensive and continuous nursing care. Team leaders on the day shift were asked to take one or two patients for whom each of them would be the 'principal responsible nurse'. During this phase of implementation, the innovation was acutally called PRN nursing. Without relinquishing any of their team leadership responsibilities, they tried to develop comprehensive care plans that would be operative 24 hours a day, seven days a week for one or two selected patients. Within a short period of time, it became apparent that the supervisory aspects of their team leader roles were all consuming; RNs had no time or energy left to concentrate on the needs of a particular patient or two. That kind of concentration would only have had the effect of short-changing all the other patients as well as reducing the team leader's availability to the team members. After a couple of months it became apparent that if staff nurses were going to be effective in providing nursing care to sick people, then their use as foremen or supervisors over large numbers of patients had to cease. The decision to try assigning 24 hours a day responsibility to all staff nurses, each one having a small case load and having her care decisions in effect even when she was not on duty seemed a worthwhile way to try to accomplish the patient care goals identified above. Within two weeks, the staff's enthusiasm had infected all of us working on 'Project 32'. The system was then dubbed Primary Nursing and the revolution was under way.

3

ELEMENTS OF PRIMARY NURSING

Primary Nursing is a system for delivering nursing service that consists of four design elements: 1) allocation and acceptance of individual responsibility for decision making to one individual; 2) assignments of daily care by case method; 3) direct person-to-person communication; and 4) one person operationally responsible for the quality of care administered to patients on a unit 24 hours a day, seven days a week.

The quality of the nursing care thus delivered to patients is determined by the performance of the individuals in the system. Performance is a result of clinical capability, sophistication of judement, organisational ability and quality of leadership, among other factors.

The quality of nursing service in a Primary Nursing system can be good or bad, comprehensive or incomplete, coordinated or spasmodic, individualised or standardised, creative or routine. Primary Nursing does not define or guarantee the quality of nursing care. As a system, it *facilitates* a very high level of quality by enabling and empowering individuals to perform at their maximum capacity. Whether they do so or not depends on them, not on the system. Thus, Primary Nursing can be in place and the quality of care still be low. It should be pointed out, however, that the quality of care is immediately apparent in this system and those who function at unacceptable levels can be immediately identified and held accountable for their performance. Unacceptable levels of performance can be dealt with appropriately *because* the levels of quality are visible.

Many people have mistakenly equated the concept of a system of care delivery with the concept of quality care. This chapter gives an explanation of the four design elements of the system; role expectations are described in the context of these elements, but whether or not they are met does not determine the presence or absence of Primary Nursing.

RESPONSIBILITY

The first element, the clear, individualised allocation of responsibility for decision making about patient care, is the heart of Primary Nursing, the essential difference between it and other systems for delivering nursing care. The Primary Nurse is responsible for deciding how care will be administered to her patients on an around the clock, continuous basis. In functional and case method, decisions are usually made by the head nurse, or charge nurse. In team nursing, decision making/care planning is the product of a team conference which is led by a team leader, and the care plan is thus the product of a group decision-making process. In Primary Nursing, decisions about a patient's care are made by the bedside nurse who has accepted responsibility for this task.

In addition to deciding how care shall be administered, she personally administers the care whenever possible. This design element recognises the fact that the person performing an activity is usually the person best able to decide how it should be done. Decentralised decision making can be defined as putting decision-making authority at the level of action. In hospitals, the action level is the bedside, and the action person, the bedside nurse. The Primary Nurse is both a planner of care and a giver of care. In commenting on the integration of these two functions one staff nurse said

> I like the freedom I'm allowed. I like the freedom of making my own decisions, deciding what my patients need. I like it because I get more involved with my patients and can learn more about them than I did in team leading. I feel much more satisfied because I have a much better understanding of the patients and all of their needs.[12]

It is essential that this acceptance of responsibility be visible to people within and outside of the delivery system. Thus, the patient, the patient's friends and relatives, the physicians, other nurses and other members of the health team must know the name of the Primary Nurse.

There are three major areas of concentration required in the exercise of this responsibility. First of all, the Primary Nurse is responsible for making available the necessary clinical information others need for the intelligent care of her patient in her absence. This means the Primary Nurse must not only be knowledgeable herself but also must be able to recognise what information is essential for the others to have and what is not. The types of areas of significant information are not defined in advance for her; it is up to each nurse to decide this on a patient-by-patient basis. In some cases, it may be the etiology or prognosis of the disease or, in others, the fact that this is a familial disease. In one case it may be the symptoms to watch for, while with another patient it may be important to know that a new form of treatment is being used. In some cases, the Primary Nurse may decide there is no clinical information of significance to be shared with her colleagues; that too is her decision to make.

Second, the Primary Nurse is responsible for deciding how nursing care shall be administered and for making that information available to other nurses in the form of instructions for care. The nursing process is useful in fulfilling this responsibility.

The Primary Nurse collects information using whatever sources are available to her, such as the patient, the chart, the physician, the patient's relatives, etc., and on the basis of the data thus collected develops a preliminary plan of care. Different hospitals provide different tools for use in data collection and writing the plan of care: nursing history forms, Kardex care plans, nursing order sheets, admission guides or whatever. Any of these can be helpful in assisting the nurse in the planning process but their design should in no way restrict the quality or quantity of data collection or the clarity with which the resulting care decisions are made. Decisions about how nursing care should be administered are of a much higher quality when the patient and his family participate in them. Deciding how and when a treatment procedure can best be performed or when hygienic care is most important to a particular patient or what time of day physical therapy is best tolerated can best be made with the full cooperation of a knowledgeable patient. Since the quality of a care decision is vastly superior under these circumstances it is incumbent upon the Primary Nurse to educate her patients so their contributions can be meaningful and useful.

Instructions left by the Primary Nurse are to be followed by others caring for her patients in her absence, unless an alteration is dictated by a change in the patient's condition. When that happens, the nurse's instructions may be modified to deal with the new situation. Otherwise, they are to be followed by the staff members who care for her patient on the other shifts, and her decisions continue in force even after she is off duty. Thus, if a Primary Nurse has written a comprehensive plan of instructions for a new diabetic that calls for his injecting an orange for the first time on a shift on which she is not working, the nurse caring for the patient on that shift should supervise, assist or teach the patient how to do the procedure.

A disagreement about how a patient should be treated or instructed must be openly negotiated and resolved but must not be fought out on the battleground of the patient's care plan. Simple differences of opinion should be easily resolved in an adult fashion by the individuals involved; serious conflicts regarding patient care may require the use of conflict resolution skills by the head nurse.

The third area of major responsibility the Primary Nurse has is discharge planning. She is then responsible for seeing to it that the patient and his family, if they will be caring for him after he leaves the hospital, have been prepared to do so safely and effectively. If the patient is being transferred to an agency that employs nurses, the Primary Nurse is responsible for transferring the necessary information that will be helpful in facilitating a smooth transition. She should tailor each discharge to each individual patient. For example, nurses in an agency or institution to which the patient is being transferred should be given relevant information in a fashion and degree of detail appropriate to the circumstances. A routine referral form may be all that is needed in one case, while for another patient a supplemental discharge summary letter may be indicated. Quite often certain information will be best supplemented by a personal phone call from the

Primary Nurse to the nurse in the nursing home or visiting nurses association. Occasionally, it may be necessary for arrangements to be made for a nurse to accompany a patient to the other institution. Hospital policies should be constructed to allow for the design of individualised discharge plans.

DAILY ASSIGNMENT—THE CASE METHOD

The second design element of Primary Nursing is the case method of assignment. 'Case method' simply refers to the way care tasks are assigned on a shift-by-shift basis, namely that one person performs all the care tasks for a particular patient regardless of the skill level of the tasks, within the limits set by that person's job description. The underlying rationale of daily patient assignments determining which care giver shall care for which patient on any given day must be the best possible matching of the needs of the patient with the abilities of the care givers available. Assignments should reflect the use of common sense.

Each person so assigned has responsibility to administer care without frequent reminders. If her job description prohibits the performance of certain required activities, she is still responsible for seeing that someone with the required preparation carries out that task. For example, an LPN who is caring for a patient receiving intravenous fluids observes the rate of flow, informs an RN when fluids must be added, and sees that this is done at the appropriate time.

Case method assignments are patient centred rather than task centred. Care activities can be grouped during one visit to a patient's room, and the hurry associated with the performance of isolated technical tasks for a large number of patients is eliminated. There is more time to talk with patients, to find out what they need or would like, to learn things about them which may affect care plans or discharge plans. In several situations where, for one reason or another, it was not feasible to implement Primary Nursing in its entirety, switching from team nursing to the case method still represented a considerable improvement. Almost immediately, the hectic, harried atmosphere characteristic of busy team nursing stations became less frantic, with a more measured pace of activities.

Criteria for patient assignments

As noted above, the most important criteria for deciding who should give daily care are: 1) the unique needs of each patient, and 2) the skills and particular strengths of the available staff members. Team nursing required the use of the most extensively prepared care giver, the registered nurse, as an overseer of less skilled, less expensive labour. It was not uncommon in such cases for the team leader to assign herself to no patients. In situations where serious staffing deficiencies left no choice the team leader would, illogically, take on an assignment of those patients who were least in need of her advanced skills. In the case method of assignment, nurses and patients are matched according to their needs and abilities, respectively. In this way, the most acutely ill patients are cared for by registered nurses, patients with intermediate degrees of illness are cared for by licensed practical nurses and, if nurses' aides are used to give direct care, it is to the least acutely ill patients.

Geography, or the location of patients' rooms in relation to each other should have little, if any, effect on assignment decisions. Admittedly, the head nurse is challenged with needing a better knowledge of her staff's abilities in order to match these optimally to patients' needs, whereas geographically-based assignments are much easier, but it is the head nurse's job to know her staff. Assignments based on patient room locations would make sense only if the top priority were to reduce the number of steps the staff nurses have to take on a given shift. However, while the assignment of patient rooms next to each other would seem to save walking time the fact is that the clustering of care activities for each patient made possible by the case method reduces the number of steps and the amount of time spent walking from one patient's room to another most effectively.

However, zones, districts or modules are enjoying a certain amount of popularity as determinants of the assignment process, despite the fact that they ultimately restrict freedom of decision making and often have a negative impact on unit morale. Such arbitrary rigidity in assigning patients results in an excessive narrowing of a staff member's awareness of all the patients on the station. Geographical assignments result in territorial attention spans. Repeated assignments to care for patients in one geographical area, although intended to enhance continuity of care, often result in the nurses honestly lacking awareness of the other patients' care needs. This in turn leads to an understandable unwillingness to pitch in and help other nurses or to answer a strange patient's signal light. Geographically grouped assignments can also result in less continuity of assignments on units where patients are frequently transferred from one room to another. Instead of districts, modules or zones, continuity of care is best maintained by having the Primary Nurse administrator care personally when she is on duty and by having all other staff members follow her care plan when she is off.

DIRECT CHANNELS OF COMMUNICATION

The third design element of Primary Nursing was developed to correct the data distortion identified previously as a problem inherent in the communication 'pyramid' of team nursing. This element provides for a direct communication channel among the nursing staff members as well as from the nurse to the patient, to the doctor, dietician, physical therapist, pharmacist, chaplain, etc. This element is simply a flattening of the communication pyramid so that important information is not filtered through a middle person; one care giver communicates directly with another care giver.

Station communications typically centre on the shift report as an essential time of information transmission. This design element calls for the care giver on one shift to report directly to her counterpart on the on-coming shift. The actual way in which the shift report is handled is not of particular importance. Tape recorders work fine for some people, and not at all for others. Some groups like walking rounds, while others have staff members moving in and out of the conference room. (Coordination may be a problem. If report begins taking twice as long as before, a change in method should be explored.) Anyone who needs to hear a report should be welcome to attend. If at all possible, charge nurses and all on-coming staff will probably want to listen to the complete report. The only irreducible requirement of this design element is simply that the caregiver on one shift must report to the person who will be caring for her patient on the next shift.

The Primary Nurse is also responsible for initiating communication directly with other members of the health team who either have information she needs or who need information she has. This means that if her patient's IV is to be maintained at 32 drops a minute throughout the time he is in diagnostic radiology, she is responsible for making sure the technician or radiologist caring for the patient during the procedure has this piece of information. Likewise, if there is some aspect of the patient's dietary management the nurse does not know or does not understand, she is personally responsible for calling the dietician to get the information. If the nurse wants to know more about the medical treatment plan she is responsible for taking the necessary steps to acquire this information; conversely, if she thus learns of information that she feels the physician should know, she is responsible for communicating it to him. In short, the Primary Nurse is responsible for getting from and giving to any other member of the health team all information which is pertinent to her patient and his needs. (One of the many pleasant corollaries of implementing this aspect of Primary Nursing is that suddenly the rest of the hospital discovers that a station staff consists of many individuals besides the head nurse, each with separate identities and unique contributions to make. The value of this to the nursing staff, and to nurses in general, is obvious.)

The role of a Primary Nurse in communicating with the patient and his family cannot be over-emphasised. As she becomes familiar with her patient's personality and his needs for knowledge about his condition, she can perform a very useful function in 1) responding to his requests for further information whenever and however it is appropriate for her to do so, and 2) interpreting his needs for additional knowledge to other members of the health team, especially physicians. Occasionally (particularly when the bureaucracy of the hospital impedes responsiveness to the patient's needs) it will be appropriate for the Primary Nurse to assume an active role as patient advocate.

Responsiveness to the patient's needs to know and enlisting his full participation in decision making is recognised as a strong and positive factor in reducing malpractice suits. Many hospitals view Primary Nursing as an important asset in reducing their potential for law suits resulting from patients' lack of knowledge. The Primary Nurse can be extremely beneficial in interpreting the patient's need for knowledge and making sure physicians and others know how much he needs and wants.

CARE GIVER AS CARE PLANNER

Because in Primary Nursing the power to decide how a patient shall be cared for is allocated to the individual personally responsible for *providing* the majority of that care, the adequacy or inadequacy of the care plan is immediately obvious to the person best qualified to decide how it can be improved. Equally important, because of this integration of the functions of care planning and care giving, the improvement can be implemented without delay.

As a result of the American Nurses Association Position Paper of 1965 many nursing departments attempted to reserve the team leader role for the baccalaureate graduate, the 'professional nurse'. The thinking was that the professional nurse would be responsible for the process in all respects except the actual implementation of the care plan. The team members, aides, LPNs and RNs with technical preparation, would be the ones to 'lay on the hands' and carry out the decisions made by the baccalaureate prepared nurse. The morale problem which inevitably follows from this arrangement is disastrous. It requires in effect that team members undergo a lobotomy each morning when they put their caps on their heads. It requires further that a given team member follows the orders of a team leader who may have had little direct contact with the patient and no firsthand knowledge of his specific care needs, and who may never herself have performed a particular procedure she is prescribing or be as able to judge its adequacy in practice as the person who actually carries it out. It should be noted too that this arrangement, aside from the morale problem it breeds, has supplied endless ammunition to those physicians who would like nurses relegated to servant status. They seize on the predictable clinical errors to which it gives rise and exhibit them as typical results of nurses' pretensions to decision-making authority, while the benefits that derive from care planning by knowledgeable care providers intelligently and logically assigned remain obscured from their view.

The decision to integrate the roles of care planner and care giver forces a different way of thinking about how to assign nurses with different job descriptions and different skill levels. Reserving the function of care planning to individuals with a particular type of education, regardless of the ability levels of others, is really a form of functional assignment. We think of functional assignments primarily as assigning such care tasks as temperature-taking to an aide, blood pressure readings to an LPN, etc. But assigning the thinking part of nursing, which is what care planning according to the nursing process is, only to individuals with certain letters after their names is part of the same functional approach to work assignments, and suffers from the same unnecessary limitations.

Although thinking and doing are integrated in Primary Nursing, the problem of assigning work according to ability still exists. The approach to this which I advocate is to match patients and nurses according to the predictable needs of patients over time and the known abilities of individuals on the nursing staff. Thus, if a well adjusted, otherwise healthy, middle aged person is admitted to the hospital for an elective appendectomy and the course of hospitalisation is expected to be uneventful, a new graduate just learning her role may be the Primary Nurse with or without close observation by an experienced RN or the head nurse. However, if the same patient expresses overwhelming fear of anaesthesia and is found to be quite hypertensive at the time of his admission, the decision might better be to assign this patient to an experienced registered nurse. Thus, the criteria for the assignment of Primary Nurses include not only a sophisticated judgment of individual nurses' abilities and interests, but also a thorough knowledge of the implications of a patient's medical condition and an early assessment and prediction of his response to hospitalisation.

Assuming that level of education does usually have an impact on level of practice and expertise, graduates of baccalaureate programmes can generally be expected to perform better with patients:

whose outcomes are not predictable;
whose care programmes are not standardised; and
whose psychological reaction to illness and/or hospitalisation is threatening their
   ability to cope with life.

Graduates of non-baccalaureate programmes can generally be expected to give adequate care to patients:

whose care programmes are standardised;
whose outcomes are predictable; and
whose psychological reaction to hospitalisation and/or illness is not threatening
   their ability to cope with life.

Experience as well as education must be taken into account when assessing an individual nurse's level of expertise in caring for various kinds of patients. Some people learn continuously through life's experiences and grow daily in their understanding and ability to cope with new situations. Others can graduate *summa cum laude* and never learn another thing in the crucible of the real world. Decisions as to who takes care of which patients should reflect sensitivity to and awareness of each individual nurse's ongoing development.

When a station implements Primary Nursing, it is realistic to expect that within a reasonable period of time all registered nurses will be able to function as Primary Nurses with their own caseloads. Of course, defining a reasonable period of time must be done by the individuals in the situation; I personally cannot imagine *any* circumstances in which that period would exceed one year. The system depends on and reflects individual qualities much more than academic degrees. One of the earliest evaluations of it came from a physician who endorsed it but pointed out that 'It makes the good nurses look good and the weak nurses stand out like sore thumbs'.

A Primary Nurse cares for her own patients on five of the 21 shifts into which the work week is usually divided. New graduates, licensed practical nurses, part-time nurses and other Primary Nurses can all be assigned to care for patients whose Primary Nurse is off duty, as Associates to the Primary Nurse. Whatever the individual's job title, or work frequency, she is expected to follow the instructions of the patient's Primary Nurse unless a change in his condition necessitates a modification of them. Therefore, on any given day a Primary Nurse may have under her care her own two, three, or four patients plus (depending on staffing that shift) one, two or three patients of a Primary Nurse who is then off. For her own patients she is continuously developing their care plans; for patients of a Primary Nurse who is off duty, she follows the instructions left on the care plan by the patient's Primary Nurse. One individual may thus be assigned as both Primary and Associate during a single shift.

Role of the head nurse

The single most critical role change necessary for the successful implementation of Primary Nursing is that of the head nurse. The skills, behaviour and attitudes that make one a successful head nurse in team nursing are different from those necessary for success in Primary Nursing. In team nursing, the successful head nurse is the one who can answer everyone's questions and solve a multitude of problems, large and small. The head nurse who knows each doctor's personal preferences, how to get a specimen sent to a lab in Timbuctoo, where extra supplies are hidden, and how best to report medication errors is a gem in any system. If in addition to all this she is able to run her floor with a minimum amount of overtime she receives another jewel in her crown. In the team nursing system the hospital world also wants her to know all about each patient's care needs, at least insofar as those needs affect the various services different individuals and departments provide. The physical therapist expects her to know how the patient is doing on bed to chair transfers, the dietician asks why the patient doesn't eat his sixth meal before bedtime, the physician wants to know whether the patient's abdomen is more or less distended today than it was yesterday and the central supply room wants her to know why this patient needs a scultetus binder instead of one of the new disposable ones. The good head nurse is the fount of all of this knowledge and the more accurately and speedily she can answer such questions, the better a head nurse she is.

Rewards for being a good head nurse are powerful in the team nursing system.

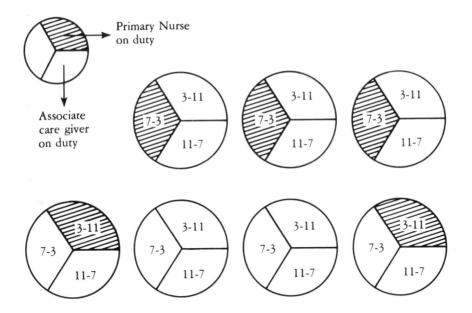

Typical Primary Nurse shift assignment. In one week the Primary Nurse works five shifts and her associates cover the other sixteen.

Most career nurses who were head nurses at some point in their past look at those years with fondness and warm feelings. The job satisfaction from being a 'good head nurse' is a unique experience. Physicians, the nursing office, and department heads are powerful reward sources. To be known as a 'good head nurse' in those circles is gratifying.

When questioned about the differences between being a head nurse in team nursing and in Primary Nursing one person said:

> My sense of satisfaction has changed. In the past it came from knowing it all when dealing with the physicians, but now it comes from seeing the staff feeling good about what they are doing and their development. It makes you feel good seeing them . . . just as they get satisfaction from seeing their patients do well, I get my satisfaction from seeing them do well.

To make Primary Nursing work, the head nurse has to turn all of those questions over to the staff nurses. Since the Primary Nurse is responsible for direct communication with all members of the health team the head nurse has to learn to refer critical questions to her. In addition to having responsibility for communication, the Primary Nurse actually has greater knowledge of her particular patients. This is often troublesome for head nurses to accept when they have a need to know more than their staff knows. Some head nurses feel insecure when they are known to have less knowledge than their subordinates. In team nursing it was, indeed, a mark of an ineffectual leader not to know the answers to everyone's questions. In Primary Nursing, however, the head nurse must recognise and respect the superior knowledge the staff has of their own patients. She has to show that respect by declining to answer questions that can best be answered by the care giver, even when she does in fact know the answers.

> Everyone is equally respected and there is no power struggle here.
> Everyone is doing patient care and making decisions and being responsible. Everyone has gone through the pitfalls of making mistakes and knowing that they did something wrong. But they also know that everybody else they work with did that too so they accept each other's mistakes.

> I think a lot of it depends on the head nurse. If the head nurse is one who just wants to maintain her power and her control over the floor it's kind of earth-shattering for her to realize that other nurses are going to be able to have the same kind of control . . . they are going to be able to go to doctors and talk to the doctors about their patient's particular problems and take care of the problems that she used to take care of. A lot of it depends on the head nurse being able to guide the floor and teach the nurses in the change-over.[13]

Many head nurses are very uncomfortable with this part of the transition. Once the adjustment to the new communication patterns has been accomplished, the rewards for head nurses begin to focus on nursing practice and the transition will proceed smoothly. They enjoy the satisfaction of watching their staff's self-image improve, their professional competence become more widely and deeply appreciated and the quality of patient care improve to the extent that patients maintain communication with them even after discharge and, if rehospitalisation is necessary, specifically request a return to the unit of *their* Primary Nurse.

The head nurse role is one of clinical leadership and continuous responsibility for the overall management of patient care. In the area of clinical leadership, the head nurse must be a teacher, the validator of decisions made by her staff, a resource person, and the quality control supervisor for the unit.

As a teacher, she is responsible for making sure that every staff nurse has the basic knowledge needed to perform safely on the unit. Whenever deficiencies are noted, the head nurse should either provide the necessary teaching personally or make other arrangements for it. (If teaching occurs without learning, then the head nurse has a personnel management problem.) Beyond basic knowledge, the head nurse ought to set the tone for the staff in striving for growing excellence by pursuing herself the knowledge that will lead to better practice. As a learner she can set a powerful example for the staff by her own continued professional and personal development.

As a validator of clinical decisions made by the staff, the head nurse must acquire the skill either 1) of agreeing with the decision and, hence, validating it, or 2) if she disagrees, of telling the staff member why and suggesting alternative approaches for the staff nurse to use in making a new clinical decision. If at this point the head nurse takes over the decision-making authority that rightfully belongs to the Primary Nurse, she will undermine the entire system. Even when a particular nurse wants a decision made for her, the head nurse must be aware of the negative effects of the usurpation of legitimate authority. Decision validation is a new skill required of head nurses in the Primary Nursing system, and time for this kind of learning must be allowed.

As a resource person, the head nurse can fully satisfy the leadership aspects of her role. Because her job is pivotal in the overall operation of the hospital, the head nurse has access to much information that staff nurses do not. Therefore, she is in a better position to know where to get different kinds of help, where particular areas of expertise are to be found and what sources are available to provide different kinds of help. When a staff nurse comes to her with a patient care or patient management problem, a good head nurse will be able to suggest four or five new alternatives for the staff member to explore in solving that particular problem.

Responsibility for the overall quality of nursing care administration on the unit 24 hours a day, seven days a week, is the responsibility that most clearly differentiates the head nurse's role from that of her staff. She must be able to evaluate the clinical nursing care decisions made by each of the Primary Nurses to make sure they are adequate, safe and, in any given circumstances, the best possible. To do this, the head nurse has to know the clinical needs and problems of all the patients as well as the strengths and weaknesses of the various members of her staff. She needs to monitor the decisions being made on a regular basis (periodic sampling techniques being quite effective). As performance weaknesses are identified, the head nurse needs to work with the staff nurse to overcome those deficiencies.

A level of supervision has been eliminated from this system, that of the 'checker upper for cheaper doers'. An implicit assumption is that individual staff members can be trusted to provide the care patients need without frequent reminders. However, if a staff member does not measure up to this assumption it is the head nurse's job either to provide corrective learning experiences or to take appropriate personnel management action.

This responsibility for overall quality of care points to an important consideration of Primary Nursing—station size. During the staff shortages of the 1960s, hospital literature reflected a growing concern about the appropriate size of a station. Many articles were written by hospital administrators and hospital architects in favour of quite large stations. (Few articles, if any, have been written by directors of nursing on this subject.) The larger the station, the more economical the staffing was the theme being played. (The expense of salaries for head nurses was thus reduced.) As a result, many hospitals expanded station size or built new, larger ones. The question of how many patients one person could care for adequately was not seriously considered as a part of the size equation as put forth by the hospital administrators and architects. In Primary Nursing, however, the importance of this factor cannot be overlooked. When the 'checker uppers' no longer exist and one person is responsible for the management of care on a continuous basis, the question of station size and number of personnel to be supervised becomes paramount. It has been my experience that 50 acute care patients are too many for one head nurse to manage effectively. The clinical knowledge requirement plus the need for familiarity with all the staff's abilities and deficiencies militate against the implementation of Primary Nursing on excessively large stations.

The head nurse as manager

If a hospital holds the head nurse responsible for the quality of nursing care administered on a 24 hours a day, seven days a week basis, authority commensurate with that level of responsibility must also be allocated. Examples of powers which the head nurse must have in order to fulfill her responsibilities include selection of personnel, allocation of resources, evaluation of performance, setting standards for the practice of nursing care, participating in the decisions about how those standards will be accomplished, and the right to terminate those who do not measure up to the standards she set. If a head nurse is not involved in the selection of personnel, her management authority is eroded. If she does not participate in the evaluation of permanent evening and night staff members, her authority over them does not exist. If she cannot terminate a staff member whose performance is unacceptable, she cannot be held responsible for that nurse's performance. Even though most head nurses have not been prepared to exercise such broad authority, it is vital that they *learn* to do so and *demand the right* to do so. The 'who and when' management decisions are of paramount importance to the structuring of a strong role for head nurses. As Jean Barrett wrote as far back as 1949:

> Good management and congenial working relationships require that no individual should be held responsible for work unless she is granted sufficient authority to prescribe how it shall be done. If she does not have this authority the responsibility for the performance must rest with someone else.[14]

All across the country, head nurses are receiving crash courses in financial management. As cost containment issues capture the minds and hearts of health industry leaders, the issue of controlling money spent has become crucial. Head nurses are being taught about salary, expense and revenue budgets. Expenditures excessively over and under the budget require explanations. This new area of responsibility can have a positive effect on strengthening the managerial role of the head nurse. However, unless it is matched by authority to make decisions about revenues and expenditures this new responsibility will become a troublesome burden and liability.

In this author's opinion one of the problems with modern hospitals is that head nurses are held accountable for areas of station operation over which they have no control. All too often this is demonstrated by a head nurse saying something like 'I'm sorry, doctor, I'll see what I can do about that missing lab report', when in point of fact she has no authority over the laboratory reporting system and, therefore, cannot really do anything about its failure. By apologising to the physician for every breakdown within the hospital system, head nurses perpetuate the myth that they have control where they actually have none. It would be far healthier for everyone concerned if head nurses were to stop apologising immediately for those system failures over which they have no control and let those who do experience the consequences of their decision-making errors.

The head nurse's role as outlined in this chapter integrates clinical and management components into a single position of strength that includes operational responsibility for competent nursing practice around the clock, every day. Primary Nursing works best where the head nurse is both a good clinician and a good manager. It flourishes in a system where decentralised decision making is the philosophy of management throughout the department of nursing.

4

THE IMPLEMENTATION OF PRIMARY NURSING

There is no one right way to do Primary Nursing. Each implementation has to be tailored to the setting in which it occurs. A step-by-step cookbook approach is not likely to result in success. The magic formula simply does not exist. In the ten years I have been involved with the system. I have managed or been a consultant to numerous successful implementations and have seen or heard about as many unsuccessful ones. The approach I am recommending in this chapter uses every bit of the real work experience I have had. It is not an easy implementation process, but it is an effective one.

The three factors most instrumental in the successful implementation of Primary Nursing are:

A. the involvement of station staff members as decision makers;
B. the use of a standard decision-making format;
C. the existence of an effective and supportive management structure.

I have chosen to start by describing the process at the station level because implementation at this level can take place without an institution-wide commitment to Primary Nursing. Later, I will describe the ideal, broader setting in which Primary Nursing flourishes, but readers should not believe that it can *only* exist in ideal institutional settings where the administrative structure is decentralised. Primary Nursing *can* be implemented in any appropriate setting using the process described in this chapter. It is not easy; it requires commitment and courage on the part of the staff. However, the results are the same. A successful implementation results in self-fulfillment of the staff regardless of whether or not the administrative structure supports the system. A successful implementation results in the establishment of relationship bonds among staff members that enable them to provide *each other* with the support not otherwise forthcoming. Risk taking is somewhat riskier, but the rewards are sweeter and the work is just as much fun.

The best way to ensure a successful implementation is to have the right people in key decision-making roles. Since this system is based on a decentralised decision-making model, the key people are those at the level of action, the staff of the nursing station (although it does help a lot if they have the support of their immediate superior). The two basic decisions are:

1. whether or not to implement Primary Nursing, and,
2. how to put the four elements of the system into effect in this particular setting.

These decisions cannot be implemented by management edict. As much as many directors of nursing would like to do just that, the results have usually been disastrous when it has been tried. There are several positive actions a management team can take to facilitate and expedite implementation; but the basic decision of whether and how to implement Primary Nursing belongs to the staff at the station.

At this level, the widest possible participation in decision making is desirable. I personally like to involve anyone who works in the station who wishes to participate, regardless of job category. (I think it far preferable to have a nurses' aide or an LPN who is worried about the loss of her own job involved in the planning process instead of outside it.) The rationale is that since all levels are affected, all levels ought to be able to participate. However, the individuals most affected by the reallocation of responsibilty, the staff nurses and the head nurse, *must* be heavily involved in the implementation process. The staff nurses, team leaders and LPNs will have a particularly important role in the implementation process and the head nurse, as formal leader of the group, is the single most important agent in the implementation process. If she is not really in favour of the system and does not support the change, it probably will not work.

Assuming that both the staff and the head nurse are agreed on the decision to implement the system, there remains another preliminary problem which has, in my experience, been the most difficult of all. The staff nurses will usually understand and welcome the difference in their new relationship with the head nurse but of far greater importance—and the very foundation of Primary Nursing—are their new relationships with each other. Hospital bureaucracies and team nursing neither require nor promote interpersonal relationships among the staff based on mutual trust and respect for one another's total nursing competence; in the absence of individualised accountability they are not particularly important among peers. However, in Primary Nursing the ability of each nurse to deal openly and honestly with others, especially in problem situations, is absolutely essential and must be emphasised from the start.

Old group identifications and territorial attitudes must be changed in the minds of staff members as they are to be changed in the new system. Night shift and day shift, RNs, LPNs and aides, 'old-timers' and 'new-comers', and so on, are no longer distinctions that have any relevance in Primary Nursing and a conscious effort to replace these with a sense of full and equal membership in the larger professional group must be cultivated. Sub-group identifications die hard, though, and every manifestation of them should be brought out into the open immediately and the healthier, constructive alternative of identification with the total group encouraged.

One sub-group that usually *is* necessary is a planning group. If the staff is small and communication lines are open and consistently effective, it may be possible to proceed without designating such a group, but stations with a large staff (over 20 people) and the usual communication problems will find that a planning group expedites the process. The selection of the group should take into account the need for representation of all shifts, categories of employees and other special interest groups. It should be small enough to be effective while large enough to represent all segments; usually eight to ten people is the best number. Members of the planning group should serve as two-way communication conduits between the rest of the staff and the group as a whole.

STEPS IN THE IMPLEMENTATION PROCESS

The standard steps of the problem solving or the decision-making process apply:

first, a definition of the problem and making a commitment to explore and evaluate the system;

second, data collection to ensure a full understanding of the system;

third, agreement (or as close to it as possible) to implement Primary Nursing;

fourth, evaluation of the effect of the system change on the delivery of nursing.

The consistent use of this process results in an inherently logical implementation tailored to the needs of the specific situation. While it is not the instant, 'magic formula' it can be relied upon to yield results.

Deciding to explore the concept of Primary Nursing is the first actual step of implementation taken by the staff. Discussions leading up to this step usually deal with a consideration of whether or not Primary Nursing is a better system for delivering nursing care than the one currently in use. If the majority of the staff is totally against *even considering* any way of improving patient care there is no point in pursuing the process of implementation. This kind of negative reaction signals the presence of serious morale problems. Most people want to improve; the absence of a desire to do so indicates the need to address other, more fundamental problems before attempting a change in system which presupposes group-wide cooperation. As one nurse summed it up:

> You really have to feel strongly about it. You really have to want to do it, otherwise as soon as something goes wrong, you can say, 'Well, we tried it but it didn't work'. You really have to want it. You have to have a strong head nurse who is going to say, 'Look, it's going to be tough to do it but it is the best kind of nursing care there is, so we have to do it.'

An effective way to start the process is to ask the entire staff to write their answers to the following questions. The written answers are not to be handed in; a verbal exchange of answers is to be encouraged, but not mandated. The more sharing, the better the process, but it must be voluntary.

Registered nurses and licensed practical nurses:
Why did you decide to study nursing?
Which parts of your job do you enjoy most?
Which parts of your job frustrate you most?
Are your original objectives being met on this job?

Support staff (aides, orderlies, technicians, etc.):
Why did you accept employment in the nursing department?
Which parts of your job do you enjoy most?
Which parts of your job frustrate you most?
Are your original objectives being met in this job?

Most people enter the nursing field because of a sincere desire to help people. Few enter for the money. Job constraints and frustrations often bury their altruistic motives. It is helpful for the staff to re-experience their earlier motivations, and discussing their answers can be a beneficial process. Again, the more sharing the better and sharing is best when it is voluntary. Some reluctance to talk about this is natural, but refusal to participate at all indicates potentially serious interpersonal relationship problems and warrants the separate attention of the head nurse, independent of the planning sessions.

If a planning group has been appointed, all members should have been in on the verbal discussion as they must have a sense of how the staff reacted. This data provides excellent background information about where people are coming from and where they feel they ought to be headed.

During this preliminary phase, the planning group should address the following questions:

What are the positive attributes of nursing care on our station?
In what ways can we improve our nursing care?
Are most of us satisfied with the results we achieve in patient care?

The answers to these questions which are valid for the group as a whole begin emerging when the personal questions asked are being discussed. Recognition of the positive aspects of care that should be preserved is as important to the success of the change process as a well developed problem statement. As the strengths and weaknesses of nursing are identified, a statement of the philosophy and the values of nursing for that station can be developed. Whether this is an informal or formal, written or spoken statement does not matter. From a synthesis of these personal assessments the group's level of professional satisfaction can be defined.

Data collection is the second step of the process. (There is not a rigid sequence to these steps; often literature about Primary Nursing appears first and then people begin talking about it.) Articles, tapes, books, personal experiences, etc. are all rich sources of information about Primary Nursing. Conversations and discussions among staff members should be encouraged. Differences of opinion, interpretation, values and meanings are useful opportunities for growth and learning. Individual staff members should be encouraged to think seriously about how this system will affect them personally. A thorough understanding of the system by each individual is important; unthinking acceptance or rejection of someone else's opinion should be pointed out and avoided. The design elements of Primary Nursing are not difficult to comprehend; ignorance due to incomprehension is a poor excuse for passive resistance. The role of staff leadership (both formal and informal) is to encourage openness and honesty. The basis for trust relationships, so helpful after Primary Nursing has been implemented, should be established during this early period of reaction to the system.

Questions quickly surface as information is acquired and digested. To the maximum degree possible, I prefer to see these questions answered on an individual, station-by-station basis. Some questions, indeed, may require a hospital-wide decision for consistency, but I prefer that recommendations even for those come from the staff instead of the management team whenever possible.

The following questions are those which most often have been asked by groups thinking of implementing this system. The questions have been grouped according to whichever of the four elements of Primary Nursing the question addresses. Many people seem to want an outside expert to answer these questions, but each department of nursing and, in some cases, each nursing staff has to participate directly in answering them to assure their relevance to that particular group. The best guidance I can give is to answer each question in terms of the patients' needs first, then nurses' needs, and to do nothing which violates your common sense.

Case method of assignment

1. What does case method of assignment mean?
2. How could it work on this unit?
3. What task limits are imposed by job descriptions? Are they necessary and definable limits? For example:
   Do LPNs pass meds?
   Regulate IVs?
   Add IV meds?
   Who should transcribe and verify physicians' orders?
   Will Aides carry a patient care assignment?

If so, who will supervise and provide back-up?

4. When the case method is used, what kinds of communication support systems are appropriate? Temperature board, intake and output summary sheet, assignment work sheet, etc.?

5. What criteria for daily assignments should be used? Rank the criteria identified according to their importance. (List should include, but not be limited to, acuity of patient conditions, skill levels, workload and room location.)

6. How will case method work on the 3 to 11 and 11 to 7 shift at the current staffing level? What effect will that have on Primary Nursing?

Twenty-four hours a day responsibility

1. What does 24 hours a day responsibility actually mean?

2. How can that be handled on this station?

3. When the Primary Nurse is off duty, under what types of circumstances should the care plan be changed? What effect, if any, will this have on her authority?

4. Do staff nurses consistently use nursing process? Is any help needed in increasing their comfort level with this activity? Are nursing histories well done when staffing permits? Are the history and care plan forms well designed? Should they be modified for Primary Nursing?

5. Is discharge planning routinely done? How about when census is down and staffing is adequate? What role do staff nurses perform in discharge planning? Is patient teaching a routine part of daily care? What kinds of support will help the staff perform this activity better?

6. Under what circumstances might it be appropriate to: a) reassign a patient to a new Primary Nurse, and b) to assign daily care to someone other than the Primary Nurse even though she is on duty?

7. Should permanent 3 to 11 and 11 to 7 nurses ever be Primary Nurses? How can communication with other members of the health team be handled?

8. If the majority of the Primary Nurses work the day shift, how can Primary Nursing be said to exist around the clock?

9. Is the clinical resource information available to the staff appropriate to its needs? If not, what should be added?

10. In addition to the full-time registered nurses, who else can reasonably be expected to function as Primary Nurses? (If part-time nurses are being considered, the question centres on how many consecutive days are worked. If LPNs are being considered, the question centres on their ability and willingness.)

Communication patterns

1. Is the principle of direct person–to–person communication well accepted by all members of the staff? By the head nurse?

2. Are there individuals uncomfortable with the thought of communicating

directly with other nurses at shift report? With doctors? With relatives of patients, or members of other departments? What kinds of assistance would help these individuals?

3. How should shift report be handled?
4. Do guidelines currently exist for presenting information at report? If not, who should develop these guidelines? Should a tape recorder be used? Walking rounds? Face-to-face report? How long should report take? Who should be present?
5. How often should patient care conferences be held? For what purpose? Who should call a conference? Who should conduct it?
6. Who should transcribe physician orders? How should a nurse be notified of new orders?

Role of the head nurse

1. How can the head nurse be most helpful to the staff in Primary Nursing?
2. How can she best monitor the quality of care being administered?
3. Should the head nurse take patients? Should she be a Primary Nurse or work as an Associate to a Primary Nurse when off duty?
4. Should there be a charge nurse with overall responsibility for station-wide decision making on each shift? Prepare a statement describing the role of the charge nurse.
5. Prepare a statement describing the role of the head nurse and Primary Nurse.

As soon as the staff have answered to their own satisfaction the first three or four questions under case method of assignment, that phase of the implementation process can be undertaken. Task limitations that exist by job description may or may not pose serious constraints on the implementation of case method. Differences in what aides and LPNs are permitted to do vary widely from hospital to hospital. (Some variations are geographical, others exist within the same community, and some, indeed, within the same hospital.) Hospitals where LPNs have traditionally administered medications and where clerical staff have already been transcribing orders will probably find little need to adjust job descriptions as they move from task-based to case-based assignments. Of all the questions listed under case method, the one about job descriptions is the one most likely to require department-wide and perhaps hospital-wide attention. Even though a station staff will not have the final authority to determine task limits set by job descriptions, their recommendations must receive careful attention and thoughtful consideration by those who will be making that decision, and deliberate communication of the staff's solidarity will help assure this.

The group's participation in answering the question about criteria for daily assignment should have an overall beneficial effect on morale. Resentment can be generated by perceived inequities in assignments. Participation in determining the criteria for assignments can provide a non-emotional forum for discussion that can lead to greater understanding and provide the opportunity to resolve old negative feelings. When everyone understands the ground rules and when those rules are applied fairly, ill feeling about workload inequities are eliminated.

Communication pattern changes can be started during the first phase of case assignment. Inadequate communication skills have been one of the largest road blocks to overcome in implementing Primary Nursing. Many individuals experience discomfort in communicating with other members of the health team, particularly with physicians. Others feel unprepared to report off at the end of the shift. Guidelines for shift report may need to be developed to help the inexperienced nurse with this communications requirement. These typically consist of a simple listing of the sequence of patient data to be followed in giving the report. Assertiveness classes have been very helpful in teaching nurses how to communicate effectively with other members of the health team (particularly physicians).

The acquisition of communication skills is an ongoing process. The two types of problems listed above are some that this author has frequently encountered. Feelings of inadequacy and apprehension due to insecurity should be identified early in the process of implementation. Changes in the communication patterns are critical to the successful implementation of Primary Nursing. Appropriate educational resources need to be made available as soon as learning needs are identified.

As the work of answering the above listed questions proceeds concrete changes are occurring simultaneously. Some typical ones are:

1. Elimination of the team leader role assignment, which has the immediate effect of adding two care givers on each day's assignment sheet.
2. Development of new criteria for assigning patients based on skills of the staff members and on the care needs of patients.
3. Expansion of duties may occur, as with LPNs learning to pass medications. Nurses' aides may realise either expansion or contraction of their patient care responsibility, depending on their particular circumstances. Clerical personnel may likewise experience changes in their roles.
4. Check lists and other systems for handling information are examined for their usefulness when assignments are based on patients rather than tasks. For example: Is a temperature sheet listing all patients' temperatures needed when each nurse takes and records the temperatures of her own patients? (Some hospitals have decided 'yes' and others 'no'.
5. Identification of clinical learning needs begins. Without exception, taking this step has always resulted in requests from the staff for additional clinical resource material. The need to know more about the sicknesses for which their patients are being treated is always experienced at this time.

The length of time different groups stay at this step varies considerably. The right length of time is however long it takes the staff to become comfortable with the workflow adjustments. This has been as short as two weeks and as long as six months. In a few cases the decision was made to stay at this level of implementation indefinitely. This is OK. When there are immovable impediments to the further implementation of Primary Nursing, acceptance of case method as the alternative choice may well be the wisest course. As case method implementation proceeds, dialogues, conversations, staff meetings, and conferences about Primary Nursing should be continuing. The more honest sharing of feelings and widespread participation in the decision-making process there is at this time, the more interpersonal relationships will be improved. This process often has the effect of tightening the group's bonds and increasing the overall cohesiveness of the staff.

The agreement to implement the major element of the system (the allocation of responsibiity) should be made when the staff is ready to do so. The third step of the process is completely taken when each patient has been assigned to a Primary Nurse. Two ways this can be accomplished are to assign all the patients at one time or to do so gradually, over a period of time. I prefer the former approach because I have often observed that a gradual implementation results in a permanently partial implementation.

This decision should be made at a point as near to a complete consensus as possible. If a few individuals are resistant they should be asked to give the system an honest try for a six month period. Most people are willing to try a new idea for at least a limited time. Anyone completely unwilling to agree to try the system even under these circumstances probably ought to be advised to transfer to another situation. Maximum group cohesiveness is highly desirable and will have a strong influence on the outcome of the effort. The earlier emphasis on group participation in the decision-making process will have laid the necessary foundation for achieving unity at this time. Cohesiveness among the different groups and shifts provides the atmosphere of support that is vitally important in the risk taking which is a part of Primary Nursing. In fact, this system involves a double risk: that inherent in any decision-making situation (if there were no chance of failure it would hardly be a decision-making situation) and that of the visible responsibility acceptance demanded by Primary Nursing. In this context, the importance of staff cohesiveness cannot be over-emphasised.

Consensus

Staff cohesiveness and decision making by consensus can be achieved in more than one way. The technique that I have used with greatest success is off duty, off premise meetings. Usually these are evening meetings scheduled far enough ahead so that necessary arrangements can be made by those who wish to attend.

Attendance at these meetings is usually very high, if not at first, certainly by the second or third session. Someone's home is the usual setting; I have probably had some 20 to 30 meetings at my own home and have attended another ten to 15 in other homes over the years. Often the first meeting is held just prior to the final decision about implementation. The agenda preparation and leadership of the discussion is usually handled by the head nurse. There is no reason, however, why these functions cannot be fulfilled by someone else on the station, or from elsewhere in the organisation.

The decision to implement may or may not be a foregone conclusion. If the decision is affirmative, the date for implementation and the steps remaining to be taken will be identified and discussed. How communications about Primary Nursing to appropriate individuals, departments and groups should be handled at this time may also be on the agenda. All of these decisions and discussions may, of course, take place in a wide variety of settings; an off duty, off premise meeting is only one of them, but it has repeatedly proved successful.

Part of the reason for its success is that such meetings are, at one and the same time, part work and part social event, and give the staff a chance to catch up on work-related as well as personal news. It is vitally important for the evening and night staffs to attend these meetings. The identity of all staff members as one group is enhanced in this way. Intershift rivalries and tensions can be dealt with much more effectively in this kind of setting as opposed to change of shift time when tempers can be short. Thus, key representatives of all shifts and all categories of workers should be urged to attend these meetings. All station personnel must know that they are or can be members of the group that is deciding how to apply Primary Nursing. Off duty, off premise meetings were used so effectively by some groups I have worked with that they became regular features of station life.

Morale ┼

Inadequate attention to tensions between sub-groups, cliques, or factions during this period can effectively impede implementation. Smouldering resentments, long-standing jealousies, excessive valuing of credentials over experience, and negative, punitive communication patterns need to be addressed and either eliminated or minimised. Unless the staff is willing to deal with differences of opinion in a supportive, honest, non-destructive manner it will be difficult, if not impossible, to establish the trust between staff members necessary to Primary Nursing. The essence of the system is one nurse with authority over other nurses for the care of her patients. That authority cannot (and probably should not) exist in an atmosphere where people do not trust one another. Unless one nurse has authority over others and her clinical competence is trusted, continuity of nursing care between shifts cannot be maintained. The participative decision-making process that has been in use throughout the implementation process will, it is hoped, have had the effect of improving interpersonal relations to the point where disagreements about approaches to patient care can be dealt with maturely and openly.

Visibility

Psychologically, the most difficult part of Primary Nursing occurs now, when the name of the Primary Nurse is put in a place where it will be visible to everyone in the system. Some hospitals use a magnetic board at the desk area to show patient location, physician's name and nurse's name. Others put the name of the nurse on the bed card alongside the names of the physician and the patient. Others put it on the front of the chart, and on the care plan. There is no one right place; the name must simply be put wherever maximum visibility will be achieved.

The success or failure of Primary Nursing often turns on how the staff feels about this phase of implementation, because deep-seated uneasiness about taking risks may surface at this stage, although it will seldom, if ever, be the stated reason for slowing down the implementation. The staff members will probably not consciously recognise this as their basic problem, and will instead cite some of the more typical problems of Primary Nursing. The most popular reason given for the system not working is inadequate staffing. Others typically include an inadequate drug delivery system, the wrong mixture of personnel, etc. A careful and dispassionate analysis of a breakdown in the system usually reveals a perceived lack of safety on the part of the staff in accepting the risks of having their names published as the individuals responsible for particular patients.

The elements necessary for group members to deal successfully with loss of anonymity and to accept the risks of visible decision making are:

1. Establishment of trust with the members of the work group, especially between day, evening, and night shifts, and between RNs, LPNs and aides.
2. Acceptance of the fact of human error and understanding that mistakes can occur at any level throughout the department of nursing.

Realistic role development

The first time a nurse tells a patient she is the Primary Nurse can, for some, be a difficult step. Support, sharing and encouragement among staff nurses can really help in getting over the rough spots. Adequate time and attention must be devoted to dealing with these feelings.

After nurses become comfortable telling patients, physicians and others about being Primary Nurses, certain role developments usually occur. These may have been anticipated by the kinds of inservice education programmes usually given to prepare nurses in advance for implementation, but I have found that no amount of formal inservice education is anywhere nearly as effective as the development that takes place spontaneously after the system has been put into practice.

This development normally involves three phases. The first is a desire to know more about the disease processes and medical programmes of the patients. Frequently, just after implementation, nurses will begin asking for medical reference textbooks and inservice programmes about the physical problems their patients are experiencing. I have frequently found at this stage that medical lectures are most effective and welcome.

The next phase centres on the development of nursing process skills. After nurses become reasonably comfortable in talking about their new roles and feel knowledgable about the physiological and therapeutic complexities of their patient's conditions, they frequently feel the need to become more proficient care planners. Accordingly, they want to become more efficient data collectors and more effective communicators of the decisions they have made.

At this point staff nurses have consistently and repeatedly requested inservice education on nursing care plans, something quite unique in my years of experience. At this point too our historical problems with nursing care plans, as described earlier, must be dealt with head-on. The accumulated guilt over years of inadequate nursing care plans must be thrown out and a new approach adopted. The care plans were not the problem; the real problem has always been lack of coordination of care. The solution which we tried to make work for years (better nursing care plans) was inadequate because their use did not require acceptance of responsibility, and the plans themselves became the goal of care, not a means to improved coordination.

In Primary Nursing, care plans serve two purposes: 1) to communicate information about a patient's problem and programme of care to others who need it and 2) to document the fact that the nursing process has been used as the basis of the patient's care. Unfortunately, before the advent of Primary Nursing, the first purpose was seldom realised in practice. Since care plans had been used during student experiences as the basis for clinical grades, their use as a professional communication tool was completely subordinated to their use as documentation. Now that many institutions are also employing them as evidence of the quality of care administered, their original documentary purpose has again become dominant, reinforced by our desires to attain professional status through the establishment of appropriate and adequate accountability mechanisms. This emphasis, however, has been matched by a continuous erosion of their usefulness as a communication tool.

Using nursing care plans primarily as communication tools between professionals tests their true value. In order to enhance their utility in fulfilling this more meaningful function, their structure, organisation and format should be streamlined; as it normally stands now they are often cumbersome, awkward and time-consuming, as well as irrelevant to daily practice. In addition, the language typically used in them is often the legalistic jargon fostered in recent years by an exaggerated preoccupation with 'nursing and the law'. Since this sort of jargon obscures the transfer of information it is self-defeating. Nursing care plans should be written as originally intended, and ought to employ the everyday language of health professionals. If they are viewed primarily as professional communication tools the staff will respond very positively to their new found uses and usefulness.

In Primary Nursing the emphasis in care plans is clear. They must contain, first, *the clinical information others need* to care for a patient and, second, *the nursing care instructions written by the Primary Nurse for others to follow* in caring for her patient when she is off duty. These two types of information are essential. It is possible to make sure other nurses know these things through means other than writing them on the care plan (the Primary Nurse can attend report around the clock, phone in each shift, or trust others to convey accurate messages verbally) but most often in Primary Nursing the care plan is the simplest effective communication tool that can be used once the necessary changes in attitude have taken place. As one staff nurse said:

> The main problem is when we get low on staff and then the problem isn't with **Primary Nursing**, it's with trying to get histories and physicals done. We know it ourselves but the care plans aren't done. It's not documented and written so we pass it along at report. And so people really are very conscientious about passing along what they know at the shift time.

When data collection, decision making and written communication of decisions are skills nurses are more comfortable with, nursing care plans improve automatically and dramatically. In Primary Nursing directors no longer have to say, 'Joint Commission is coming' in order to assure the writing of care plans because it becomes demonstrably advantageous to the individuals using them to do so.

The third phase of role developments in Primary Nursing is the acquisition of communication techniques that enable a nurse to interact more effectively with physicians, relatives of patients and other members of the health team. Again it is fruitless to try to teach these skills until the other phases of role development have been addressed. Until the Primary Nurse is really convinced that she knows enough (about the patient, the disease, the nursing care, family, relatives or whatever) to deserve the respectful attention of others, she may be unwilling or unable to learn how to articulate her patient's needs to those who need to know. The most troublesome aspect of communication for most nurses is learning 'how to talk to God'—the physician. It is not accidental that many nurses feel that this is primarily *what head nurses are paid to do*, but in Primary Nursing this is a 'hang up' they will have to get over. Courses in communication, such as assertiveness training programmes, can enforce a nurse's self-confidence, thus enabling her to take the risks sometimes inherent in direct communication with some physicians. Group support and encouragement are also important in helping the more reticent nurses develop these skills.

These three phases of development: 1) increased knowledge of medical problems; 2) enhanced nursing process skills and 3) the ability to communicate effectively usually follow one another in a natural progression. Some nurses may need more help with certain developments than others. Nursing administration needs to recognise and accept the fact that the individual nurse is responsible for initiating her own growth and development, but should be ready to provide appropriate education resources and psychological support as necessary to facilitate that development.

As this third step in the implementation process—the agreement to and commencement of the 'trial run'—gets underway, no great expectations should be laid on the staff. I personally view this as a time of adjustment when the staff have to sort out for themselves what they want to say to patients, relatives and physicians about their new role responsibilities. Care plans, beautiful histories, and elaborate discharge plans can all come later. It is enough at this stage for the nurses to deal with their new visibility and the great challenges and opportunities of their new professional relationships.

Evaluation is the final step in the process. Initially, an informal evaluation is appropriate and adequate. Subjective responses to the change by both staff and patients will be of the greatest value in judging its genuine success.

After the system has been in effect for at least six months, whether or not its original goals have been met should be determined. A simple and effective way to accomplish this is to reissue the questions the staff were asked to answer at the beginning of the implementation process. Usually the planning group is re-formed for this task, and its members collect and summarise the answers (which may be either written or verbal). A report to the whole staff summarising individual staff members' responses to the four groups of questions can then be made. If the implementation has been wholly successful, this will be a very affirmative experience. The following are some typical reactions:

> I just think it's really neat to have a job that gives you the kind of satisfaction that I've gotten from my relationships with primary patients.

> I'm treated more like a professional person in Primary Nursing, say 80% or 90% of the time, than I ever was in team nursing.

> Here on our floor Primary Nurses are promoting patient care and themselves as professional people and everybody is beginning to recognize that. Primary Nurses really care about patients and *are* more professional.

> I think Primary Nursing has actually caused the team of the doctor

and the nurse to work better together. We're a lot closer today and I think the doctors really do respect us a lot more. I can't believe how many times the doctor now discusses things with me.

The hard core of the evaluation must be the staff's perception of its success or failure. If difficulties still exist with the implementation of Primary Nursing, this evaluation process will serve to focus attention on the problem so that it can be defined and solutions sought by appropriate staff members.

At the very minimum, the evaluation requires the participation of all members of the nursing staff. A much wider assessment is often made in which the reactions of patients, physicians and other members of the health team are sought. These can be acquired in interviews, by questionnaire or by the solicitation of testimonials. In many hospitals the approach is much more formal, but regardless of its design the subjective opinions of the staff must be solicited and the effect they perceive the system to have had on their patients must be determined. It is the obligation of each and every person entrusted to care for the sick to make sure that that care is being rendered in the best way possible. Thus, whatever else it may include and whoever participates in it, the evaluation of the system must ultimately be made in terms of its impact on patients.

MANAGEMENT AND PRIMARY NURSING

The implementation process described in the preceding chapter was a more or less isolated phenomenon. It can occur once within a given hospital, or it can occur repeatedly; it can remain a localised experiment or become the foundation of an entire hospital's care system. There are many factors that determine how widespread the implementation of Primary Nursing will be in any given institution. The three most important are: 1) the organisational theory on which the existing administrative structure is founded; 2) the attitude of management towards Primary Nursing; and 3) the functions of management in the implementation process.

ORGANISATIONAL THEORY AND ADMINISTRATIVE STRUCTURE

The organisational theory that provides the best foundation for Primary Nursing is decentralised decision making. As illustrated in previous chapters, it means simply the granting of decision-making authority to those at the level of action, who are in the best position to judge the adequacy and efficacy of the decisions they make. Decentralisation of this authority has the effect of flattening hierarchies. It recognises the value of individuals within all levels, putting them in control of their own actions and (to a somewhat lesser extent) the environment in which those actions take place. Each individual is answerable for the consequences of his actions; accountability is the flip side of the responsibility coin.

In *People or Personnel* by Paul Goodman[15] the difference between centralised and decentralised decision-making management philosophies is explained and the types of institutions or organisations that ought to be organised around the different management theories are categorised. He recommends centralised management decision making in institutions or organisations where the product of the functions performed is inanimate and where the tasks used to accomplish the functions are repetitive, mechanistic, automatic, and predictable. In institutions or organisations where the product is a human being, however, and the tasks used to accomplish the functions are neither repetitious, automatic nor predictable, he recommends the use of decentralised decision making. The human being in the hospital is never perfectly predictable and Goodman goes on to say specifically that such institutions ought to be organised around the theory of decentralised decision making.

There are three elements in the theory that need to be taken apart, examined separately as they affect each level of authority in the hierarchy of a department of nursing, and then reassembled into a cohesive administrative structure. These three elements are:

1. The clear allocation and acceptance of responsibility for decision making.
2. The delegation to an individual of authority which is commensurate with her authority.
3. The establishment of mechanisms of accountability so that the quality of the decisions that have been made can be evaluated.

The absence of these three elements in the hierarchy of the department of nursing will deter the implementation of Primary Nursing.

In Primary Nursing decentralisation means bringing decision making to the bedside. A nurse needs and is given responsibility for the nursing care received by a patient around the clock, seven days a week. She is authorised to direct the actions of other nurses who care for her patients when she is not there, which presupposes their respect and trust of her as essential ingredients in their interpersonal relationships. Mechanisms of accountability therefore need to be established so that the quality of her decisions as Primary Nurse can be examined to determine whether or not good clinical judgement is being used.

Currently, the head nurse in most hospitals provides whatever accountability there is in the system. However, quality assurance programmes are being developed in some hospitals that enable a staff nurse's decision-making process to be measured against standards of practice that have been established by other staff nurses. The development of these programmes based on standards of practice set by peers elevates our practice to a higher level of professionalism than it previously had. Peer review without being able to identify single decision makers is impossible and therefore necessitates decentralisation of decision making to the staff nurse level. It can thus be the first step in the development of a professional practice of nursing within the bureaucratic setting of the hospital.

The importance of a consistent approach to decision making throughout the administrative structure of the department cannot be overemphasised. In Primary Nursing, staff nurses are being asked to take the risk of visibility in their decision making. If the same degree of visible responsibility acceptance does not exist in the higher levels of the hierarchy, the staff nurses are likely to feel vulnerable on the one hand, and to lack trust and confidence in their superiors on the other. If individuals in superior positions will not accept, with visibility, the risks of making mistakes in management decisions, how can the staff nurse be expected to accept the risks of mistake making in clinical practice? It is very important that the responsibilities of all levels of the hierarchy are clarified and that authority is delegated accordingly. A good test of whether or not there is clear understanding of levels of responsibility and authority is to ask individuals to describe their own jobs in these terms, as well as the jobs of their immediate superiors and subordinates. If people are holding positions that they cannot describe in a way that others can understand, then a major position definition and clarification effort is called for.

A centralised decision-making structure should be decentralised in order to support the implementation of Primary Nursing. It is difficult (not impossible, but very difficult) for it to be successfully implemented when management decision making remains highly centralised. A reasonable timetable (not longer than six months) should be targeted for this reorganisation process.

An administrative structure that supports Primary Nursing must be assessed according to two criteria. The first is the degree of congruity between responsibility, authority and accountability at all levels of authority within the superstructure and the second is whether or not 24 hours a day responsibility for patient care exists at appropriate levels within the organisation.

There are only three or four natural levels of authority within any department of nursing from bedside nurse to director of nursing. The first is the Primary Nurse who has responsibility and authority for the care of a group of patients and the second is the head nurse who has responsibility and authority over the quality of care administered to an entire group of patients. In large hospitals there is usually a third level, a position of many titles. Here, for the sake of simplicity, I will just call it the 'middle management level'. The fourth level of authority within the department is, of course, that of the director of nursing who is responsible and has the authority and is held accountable for the quality of care administered throughout the institution by all members of the nursing department at all times.

To determine whether or not responsibility, authority and accountability are properly matched at the various levels of the department of nursing, a few key questions can be asked. For example: 1) Will other nurses follow the care plan of the Primary Nurse? If the Primary Nurse does not have authority over the nurses who care for her patients in her absence, then she cannot be held responsible for the quality of care a patient receives on a 24 hours a day basis. 2) Does the head nurse take the blame from a physician when a lab report is not on the chart, thus implying that she can be held responsible for something over which she has no authority? Not until the head nurse designs the lab reporting system will it be appropriate for her to accept the blame for its failure. 3) Can the supervisor of a particular area select a head nurse on her service? 4) Does the director of nursing need to ask permission from the hospital administrator or chief of the medical staff in order to implement Primary Nursing? If she does not have the authority to develop improvements in the delivery system used for nursing care she cannot legitimately be held responsible for its quality. Honest answers to these questions will help indicate the degree of congruence between responsibility and authority.

The second criterion is the clear allocation of 24 hours a day responsibility at the

57

head nurse and middle management levels of a department to ensure that adequate continuity between the shifts is successfully maintained. This is an area where lip service and reality are often inconsistent. If the head nurse does not have primary responsibility for the evaluation of the permanent 3 to 11 and 11 to 7 floor personnel, then she does not have 24 hours a day responsibility for the floor. The importance of this criterion cannot be overemphasised.

A special word is in order about the middle manager, the congruence of whose authority and responsibility is often the most out of line. Most commonly called the supervisors, they have a range of titles that runs the gamut from director to coordinator. Over the past ten years, this role has perhaps changed the most (or at least been threatened the most) and is still the least clearly defined. The dichotomy between administration and clinical practice is felt most exquisitely by individuals in this position. They are continually given more responsibility for administration, and yet many institutions seem to expect them to maintain a high degree of clinical expertise as well. So often they are the individuals called by other nurses when a special clinical problem requires expert handling. But in fact they are often the last to know of advances in medical technology because they are so preoccupied with administrative problems. (It is only in the past ten years that people have stopped expecting the director of nursing to step into complex clinical situations as the in-house expert. Most directors no longer even wear uniforms.) Changes in others' expectations of middle managers have, unfortunately, gone in one direction only: an increase in administrative involvement with no lessening in expectations of their clinical skills. This has often left these middle managers the most frustrated and insecure in the nursing family. Nevertheless, their attitude towards Primary Nursing is of importance second only to that of the head nurse, whose successful leadership in implementing Primary Nursing will often depend on the middle manager's support and a tolerant attitude towards the risk taking of decision making.

THE ATTITUDE OF THE MEMBERS OF THE MANAGEMENT TEAM

The second vital factor affecting implementation of Primary Nursing is the attitude of the management team. If its members start out with a firm belief that most nurses want to take good care of their patients, and if they adopt an attitude of support without pressure, the implementation process will be greatly facilitated and its chances for complete success vastly enhanced.

The adoption by the management team of a philosophy of support without force is of fundamental importance to the system. Primary Nursing cannot be implemented by management edict; it must be implemented by the staff of a station. This is often difficult for individuals in positions of authority to accept. For me personally it was extraordinarily difficult since my belief in Primary Nursing knows no boundaries. Since 1969, my life has been dedicated to the implementation of this system but I have had to accept, albeit reluctantly, the fact that I cannot just *make* nurses into Primary Nurses. That acceptance has been reinforced by the recognition that there are certain types of people who, if they are pressured into this system against their will, can subtly (and sometimes not so subtly) sabotage it in ways that will endanger not only its success but patient safety as well. The only way I know to avoid this kind of aggravating and destructive behaviour is to insist on these individuals' participation in the decision-making process. This will help make their actions public and their responsibility for them visible, and it will also help the individuals become more conscious of their own motivations. The important thing is that they come to see their participation as voluntary, even if it is only on a trial basis.

In my Preface I expressed my strong belief that virtually all nurses are motivated by a sincere desire to give good nursing care. This belief is essential among managers because of two important attitudes to which it gives rise. The first is that since nurses *want* to give good nursing care, few controls are necessary to prevent willful wrongdoing. Excessive use of management control mechanisms communicates to the staff an expectation that if not controlled they will perform in undesirable ways. This negative approach by management results in people feeling as if they are treated like little children, which encourages them to act that way.

The second is an attitude of tolerance toward human error. The fear of committing errors in the treatment of patients has led us into thinking of mistake making as aberrant or unnatural. Although a supreme being is presumed to be the only entity to whom we may attribute infallibility, the profession of nursing has not learned how to deal effectively with the simple, basic reality of human fallibility. From its beginning nursing has dealt with human frailty by punishment. (One wonders why society keeps trying to use punishment to control behaviour when such great evidence of its ineffectiveness surrounds us daily.) When nursing was task-oriented the nature of a mistake was quite different to what it is now that we are judgment-oriented. The nature of making a procedural mistake is quite unlike making a mistake in clinical judgment. The traditional swift and severe punishment for the former has impeded our ability to accept the mistake making inherent in the exercise of clinical judgment.

Why is mistake making inherent in this kind of judgment? Clinical nursing judgment is used to solve problems the patient presents based on the knowledge and the experience the nurse brings to the assessment of the situation. The basic steps of the decision-making process are used by the nurse and the activity is called 'the nursing process'. What we have failed to deal with in teaching nursing process is the reality that a nurse will usually have to make a decision about a problem *before* she has had time to acquire all the relevant information. This means that at least some of the time a wrong decision will be made because the information on which it was based was *inadequate*. We foster the myth that decision making is based on adequate data collection, but in the real world there is seldom time to do the literature search, thorough family interview, complete physical assessment, etc., required for completely adequate data collection. Clinical decision making must consequently admit to the possibility of error. But our knee-jerk reaction to any mistake has been punishment; our earliest reaction was to expel the wrong-doer. By the late 1940s and 1950s a student nurse who had committed an error was forced to appear in the hospital without her cap. Today, evaluations, audit reports, conferences and incident reports are sometimes used as a more subtle form of punishment.

A management team must deal with the emotional backwash of this punishment-oriented heritage. As already described, one of the most serious impediments to the successful implementation of Primary Nursing is the pure fear staff nurses feel when confronted with the requirement that their names appear on the front of their patient's charts. The initial response is frequently 'My God, he'll know who to yell at'. Members of the management team must deal openly with this problem and discuss their attitudes towards mistake making. A good exercise to start with is for each member of the management team to discuss a serious error in practice she committed in her first staff nurse position. This telegraphs the important message to the bedside nurse that management acknowledges, understands and accepts the risk-taking element of decision making. If the superiors have taken risks and admitted to human errors the Primary Nurse will feel safer and the atmosphere in which the system is being tried out will be healthier.

The two factors affecting the ease with which Primary Nursing can be implemented—the theories of organisation most conducive to its success and the most desirable attitudes on the part of management—are certainly important to the final outcome, but it should be noted that they are not essential. I have seen the system implemented in settings where the atmosphere, especially at the upper levels, was not at all hospitable. Primary Nursing can be implemented in spite of this; it simply requires more courageous staff nurses.

FUNCTIONS OF MANAGEMENT IN IMPLEMENTING PRIMARY NURSING

Once agreement has been reached to try out Primary Nursing—whether or not the decision has been unanimous, or made by a group of staff nurses, or by individuals higher up in the nursing administration hierarchy, and whether or not the theoretical basis of the organisation and the attitude of management towards the experiment are favourable—individuals at the management level must take certain steps if they wish the system to have a fair trial. The following are the most effective facilitative mechanisms I have seen used in various hospitals:

1. Internal assessment of the effectiveness of the administrative structure.
2. Appointment of a central committee for Primary Nursing.
3. Appointment of an individual to coordinate implementation.

4. The establishment of a Primary Nursing advisory council.

Putting these mechanisms into effect calls for the contributions of various managers.

The role of the director of nursing

The internal assessment of administrative efficacy has been discussed previously, in the last chapter and in the context of organisational theories. It is an area in which the director of nursing can most effectively exert her leadership by seeing to it that necessary preconditions are met:

1. Administrative support of the concept of continuous operational responsibility, clearly allocated so everyone knows who is responsible for what and when.
2. The matching of responsibility with a commensurate degree of authority for individuals at all levels of the department.
3. A philosophy of tolerance in regard to (reasonable) errors in clinical judgment, sufficient to permit necessary risk taking.

The director of nursing must not only see that these conditions exist but must also be able to articulate them to the entire department as an official philosophy, in the fulfillment of which individuals can expect administrative support.

The central committee for Primary Nursing

The appointment of a central committee to facilitate implementation on a department-wide basis has been beneficial. Members should include people in key management positions (day, evening, and night may be appropriate), some staff nurses, as well as members of the inservice education department. The chairperson of this committee should be selected for her knowledge and understanding of the entire department of nursing, the hospital as a whole, and the pockets of power that exist within the hospital community. It is important that this chairperson is seen as an agent of the director of nursing (assuming, of course, that the director of nursing supports the implementation of Primary Nursing).

The functions of this committee should include the following:

1. Identification of administrative changes necessary to support Primary Nursing.
2. Recommendation of departmental changes below the administrative level necessary to support the system of Primary Nursing.
3. Identification and dissemination of literature and information about other resources which will help staff at all levels understand and contribute to the implementation of the system.

Examples of activities this committee might perform are:

A review of the statement of departmental philosophy and objectives to evaluate its appropriateness to Primary Nursing.

A review of all other departmental and hospital policies affecting the nursing department to determine their appropriateness to Primary Nursing. Inconsistencies (e.g., use of the title 'team leader') should be ironed out through liaison with other departments.

A review of all nursing procedures to determine their appropriateness under the new system.

A review of job descriptions and their rewriting to make them consistent with the requirements of Primary Nursing.

The Primary Nursing central committee may appropriately be empowered to revise, rewrite or establish the statements of policy, procedure, job descriptions, etc. In many hospitals, though, standing committees already exist for these purposes, in which case it is better for them to carry them out. In practice the central committee's main function will be to assess the compatibility of the existing administrative systems with the principles of Primary Nursing.

The Primary Nursing system coordinator

Some hospitals (including two in which the author was Director of Nursing) have found it useful to designate someone as 'Primary Nursing coordinator' or 'Primary Nursing liaison' (or something similarly descriptive). Usually, one RN can handle this function as an additional assignment over and above her regular tasks and responsibilities (although it may be necessary on a short–term basis to reallocate some of her job responsibilities to make time for the new task). While not absolutely necessary it makes a great deal of sense for this coordinator to be chairperson of the Primary Nursing central committee as well. That way, there is one clearly visible person within the organisation who serves as a resource to individuals at any level interested in pursuing the concept of Primary Nursing. The individual selected must always be someone in a position of authority that reflects a high value in the organisation. It may be a nurse from the inservice education department or someone with special project or research and development responsibilities, or the nurse with primary responsibility for coordinating discharge referrals. The other responsibilities that this individual holds are not of particular importance. What is of primary importance is that she is well respected by all levels of the nursing staff and is seen as one who understands head nurses and, especially, the station staff.

Both the Primary Nursing coordinator and a majority of the members of the central committee are likely to be drawn from middle management levels. It is entirely appropriate for the director of nursing to expect individuals at this level to deal personally with the issues raised by Primary Nursing. Lack of support at this level can be a sufficient deterrant to prevent its implementation in the areas over which one such individual has influence. If Primary Nursing becomes an accepted goal of the department of nursing then it is reasonable and proper for the director of nursing service to expect support for the concept from the individuals in middle management positions. Sabotage of a department goal is not to be tolerated.

Primary Nursing advisory council

Another positive mechanism to facilitate the implementation of Primary Nursing is the establishment of a Primary Nursing advisory council. Historically, this council has developed as a loosely organised staff nurse/head nurse meeting where individuals already doing Primary Nursing and those considering it can discuss, *in the absence of their superiors*, the problems and solutions, successes and failures they are experiencing or anticipate experiencing in the new system. (If there is a Primary Nursing coordinator she too would normally attend sessions of this council, but not in a managerial capacity.) With its primary emphasis on the mutual sharing of experiences the greatest benefit of this council is self-growth through self-help. Since it is not a formal committee of the hospital or department *per se*, its meetings can be kept as informal as participants like. They seem to work best when nursing administration provides a time, place and advance notification, but it should not attempt to direct the meeting, select the people who attend, or hand down solutions to the problems expressed. Ideally, these solutions will come as a natural by-product of the sharing process. Solutions that require administrative actions can be brought to the attention of nursing administration by the adivsory council in the form of recommendations, which must receive careful and serious consideration and prompt action from whoever is designated to act on them: the Primary Nursing central committee, the Primary Nursing coordinator, or in many instances, the director of nursing.

To summarise, there are four positive steps that can be taken by a central nursing administration to support and facilitate the successful implementation of Primary Nursing. These are 1) an internal review of administrative structure; 2) the establishment of a Primary Nursing central committee charged with seeing that necessary department-wide changes are made to enhance departmental support for the concept of Primary Nursing; 3) the establishment of a Primary Nursing coordinator or implementor to help keep the implementation process moving; and 4) the establishment of the Primary Nursing advisory council to serve as a forum in which staff nurses and head nurses can share their experiences with the new system.

POPULAR MYTHS ABOUT IMPLEMENTATION

A few words are in order about approaches to implementation which, after being tried, have been found inadequate. One of these, which this author and others have used with little long-term success, is the establishment of a pilot station. The thinking behind experimenting on a smaller scale seems valid on the surface, but repeated experience with this approach has led me to discourage its use in any hospital that is seriously considering widespread implementation of the system.

When people are facing a change as pervasive as that from team to Primary Nursing, it seems desirable to localise the potential negative effects as much as possible. The risk of failure is not as frightening when it is restricted to a carefully controlled setting. It is assumed that under these circumstances any mistakes made in the implementation process can be more easily corrected, and that others can learn from these mistakes and avoid repeating them. However, these assumptions are founded on the flawed belief that Primary Nursing will thrive when it is imposed and controlled from above. As I have emphasised repeatedly, the system is likely to succeed only when a group of nurses who work together plan the implementation. If the staff of two, three, four or more units wish to plan concurrently, there is no reason why they should not do so. Since every staff has the right to decide the question for itself, an attempt to implement the system hospital-wide can be too unwieldy and as unlikely to succeed as a specially designated pilot station. Overall coordination of a multiple-station implementation is not an excessively difficult task. What matters most is that the first station or stations to implement Primary Nursing shoud select themselves.

The timing of implementation cannot be controlled by the director of nursing or any other individual. Primary Nursing should occur when people feel themselves ready to make the necessary changes required for the system to be put in place. I have visited hospitals where implementation institution-wide is awaiting the collection of before-and-after data from a pilot station while the staffs of other stations have been eminently ready to implement the system and have felt extremely frustrated with the enforced wait. Meanwhile, nurses on the pilot station feel as if they are living in a goldfish bowl, becoming increasingly fatigued and anxious. All in all, the establishment of a pilot station is an 'unnatural' approach to implementation, the possible advantages of which are outweighed by the likely disadvantages.

Another popular but ultimately counterproductive approach to implementing Primary Nursing is the prior establishment of a set of *selection criteria* according to which participants in the experimental programme will be picked. The underlying assumption seems to be that Primary Nurses have special characteristics, qualifications, educational preparation, or personality attributes that make them different from the average staff nurse. The inescapable destructive effect this has on morale in the nursing department cannot be overemphasised. A corollary of this assumption is that some of the individuals currently employed on the implementation station will be found unqualified to administer nursing in the new system. While criteria are being established and the selection process is getting under way the effect on personal relationships and morale in general is profoundly negative. Nothing is more likely to undermine the cohesiveness of a closely knit work group than being threatened from outside by the elimination of some of its members and the addition of new ones.

I am not suggesting that everyone employed in a particular situation will necessarily be able to perform satisfactorily in Primary Nursing. I stress again, though, that an effectively functioning group which has made a conscious decision to implement Primary Nursing should be recognised as the single appropriate milieu for the experiment. If any individual within the group is unable (or, more usually, unwilling) to make a successful adjustment to the new delivery system, the situation can be corrected after Primary Nursing is underway. It has been my experience that with the proper educational opportunities, and strong professional leadership, any individual in a care giving role finds the Primary Nursing system the most comfortable and rewarding way to carry out her job responsibilities.

Finally, there is the myth that Primary Nursing can be taught to nurses before the system is implemented so that on day one of an implementation everyone has been 'adequately prepared' to function in the *role* of Primary Nurse. This misjudgment has caused enormous amounts of frustration and a deep sense of futility in those trying to design a fool-proof implementation plan—not to mention those who are supposed to carry it out. The truth is that until the system changes the role cannot develop. People cannot learn how to perform on a more professional level of nursing in a setting that rewards only bureaucratic competence. If they could, they would have done so a long time ago. The unique role of the Primary Nurse must develop naturally and, during this process, the appropriate function of leadership is to provide educational resources and other support as needed. It is not to assess, identify, define and evaluate those needs, but simply to provide adequate resources. The role will then develop naturally and the truly professional nursing practice dreamed about by millions of nurses over the years will become the everyday reality of patient care.

⑥

PRACTICE IMPLICATIONS

EDUCATIONAL IMPLICATIONS

There are two major educational implications of Primary Nursing: the use of Primary Nurses as teachers, and the place of Primary Nursing in the curriculum.

The clinician/teacher method of nursing education is still considered by many (including the author) to be a superior teaching process. When nursing education and service were separated, use of this model disappeared, and the problems created by the loss have been serious and to a large extent unsolvable. Joint appointments of faculty who are both clinicians and teachers hold some promise of reintegrating education and service. But insofar as such appointments currently exist their usefulness is very limited, particularly at the level of basic education, and they are not sufficient to make the clinician/teacher model universal in undergraduate programmes.

The proposal I am outlining here recognises the value of increasing joint appointments and suggests that Primary Nurses, employed by a hospital, be used in a productive way as clinician/teachers for basic nursing education. Consistently positive results have supported my belief that patient presentation by Primary Nurses can, in a relatively short period of time, greatly enhance a student nurse's knowledge of complicated interrelated factors of patient care. A ten to fifteen minute presentation of a diabetic patient that focuses on the interrelated aspects of care in that complicated disease process is a far more effective use of a student nurse's time than an hour spent giving a diabetic patient a bed bath. It is unrealistic to expect classroom-based faculty to be able to teach a comparable level of clinical judgment. The Primary Nurse is the most logical one to prepare the students for the real complexities of professional nursing practice. Creative and innovative ways to tap this knowledge and make it available to student nurses should be explored by those who are responsible for the education of future nurses.

The curricular implications of Primary Nursing are profound. Teaching decision making is no mean task. The majority of Primary Nurses practising today must learn this skill on the job. Other professionals acquire it as part of their education; it is appropriate for nurses to do so also.

Decision making cannot be taught in a laboratory. If it could, teaching hospitals would never have been needed for medical education. In order to teach it effectively there must be three risk takers: a faculty member, a student and a patient (whose share of the risk is, ideally, minimal). This is true for both medicine and nursing, the only difference being that medicine has always recognised the essential priority of professional decision making.

Nursing education has not placed a high value on independent decision making by practitioners. Student nurses do not 'carry a case load' with any degree of independence even in the final stages of their preparation. Many schools still teach students how to perform as team leaders, but that role actually requires little or no understanding of problem solving or decision making. For example, as team leaders many students are still taught to collect 'all the necessary data' before making a decision about a patient's care needs. To do this at all thoroughly requires unrealistic amounts of time and consequently one finds care decisions not being explicitly made because not enough data was collected. In the real world, besides basic clinical decision making skills, students need to learn the realities of priority setting and judicious corner cutting or they will never be able to make important decisions on an hour-by-hour basis during times of busy workloads—a failure which distresses both student and patient.

There are two areas of decision making required of a care giving nurse. The first is deciding how to care for a particular patient and the second is coordinating such care for a number of patients. Clinical decision-making ability and management decision-making ability are both called for. Managing a case load of patients requires planning, including priority setting, performing the care and evaluating its effectiveness. In order to accomplish this, faculty and student nurses need to acknowledge the fact that decisions must be made in spite of incomplete data collection. Seldom does real life allow one the luxury of collecting all of the relevant data before making any sort of decision; judgment based on knowledge and experience is relied upon. This is precisely the case in nursing: informed judgment must be brought to bear in situations where a decision must be made before all the data are available. The skill to be taught then is the exercise of sound judgment (the educated guess) based on whatever facts are ready to hand. Student nurses need to learn this skill by seeing it in action, although equal care should be taken that a faculty member is not at their elbows continuously during this learning process; it then becomes the faculty member's judgment that is being used, and the student will be working to achieve approval from the teacher rather than working to solve the patient's presenting problem. In carefully controlled settings then, clinical decision making must be learned first by observing it and increasingly by practising it.

Nurses who have been in practice for a few years have extraordinary skill in patient care decision making.

> I remember in my delivery room experience being awed by the old
> time delivery room nurses' knowledge of when to call a doctor. Not

only could they predict the speed of an individual patient's dilation with unerring accuracy but they also knew how long it took each physician to travel from home to hospital or from office to hospital and manage to place the call at exactly the right time so that the doctor arrived precisely five minutes before delivery. Great skill went into making these judgments. In Primary Nursing, hopefully, that level of decision-making sophistication can be directed at patient care decisions instead of physician care decisions.

Educational curriculum experts and students of learning theory can build opportunities for unsupervised clinical decision-making experiences into the educational process, starting with basic and simple cases and gradually increasing the complexity to the greatest extent possible.

Clinical decision making in the hospital, whether by a student or experienced nurse, requires a knowledge of disease and a knowledge of human beings. Knowledge of the patient cannot be acquired in the classroom setting; it cannot even be acquired in short spurts of clinical exposure on a patient unit. Clinical decision making in nursing must be based on the nurse's firsthand knowledge of the sick person and this knowledge can best be acquired through the establishment and maintenance of a relationship over time. Thus, before students should be expected to make independent clinical decisions, the curriculum must be adjusted to permit them opportunities to establish therapeutic relationships with patients. This cannot be accomplished in a few hours a day, a few days a week; Primary Nursing requires that curricula be adjusted accordingly. Time must be allowed so that clinical decision-making skills can be learned in a relatively independent fashion. Faculties have to learn to 'let go' of their students just as head nurses have to learn to 'let go' of their staff nurses when Primary Nursing is implemented. The art of 'letting go' may actually help faculty members recognise the strength and weaknesss of the educational programme better than any paper and pencil tests could.

Management of a number of cases simultaneously is another important skill needed in Primary Nursing. Setting priorities to get work done is a common enough concept in nursing service. Workload expansions and contractions inevitably occur without commensurate staffing adjustments, and since extra staff cannot be added to cover all such situations nurses need to learn how to decide which of their patient's needs will be met and which ones will not. Nurses may then feel less guilty about the fact that all patients do not receive all the care that they could simply because there are not adequate resources available. Nurses seem usually to be plagued with a tremendous sense of guilt about their inability to do everything for their patients. This is quickly transformed into anger and frustration, and enormous amounts of energy are wasted because of 'short staffing'. Nurses in hospitals today need to realise that there will never be as much help as they need or would like on their units and that the necessary priority decisions about how their time will be spent should only be made by them. Physician needs are often in competition with patient needs for nursing attention. Students should be taught that patient care needs come first and physician needs second. Once priorities have been set, nurses have to be realistic and stop feeling guilty about all the care they were unable to give, and learn instead to enjoy the accomplishments of delivering that care which is really essential.

The ability to establish, maintain and terminate the therapeutic relationship is another learning need made visible by Primary Nursing. Never a strong component of nursing education, this skill was ignored when this author was a student. We were taught not to get involved with our patients, to maintain a professional aloofness. Sister Madeline's work on commitment as an essential component of professional nursing helped pave the way for the kind of caring relationships that characterise the successful implementation of Primary Nursing.[16] The need for such relationship skills is more widely recognised now but the fact that many nurses are still very uncomfortable in this regards indicates that it should receive increased attention. No one is born with a complete and intact set of interpersonal skills; they must be learned and, until they are, it should be recognised that their lack is an educational lack, not an inadequacy in the nurse or in the system of Primary Nursing.

THE MEANING OF CLINICAL SPECIALISATION

For years the profession of nursing has been trying to identify logical parameters of clinical specialisation around elements of nursing care rather than medical diagnoses. Nevertheless, clinical specialisation in nursing still follows the medical model closely. Thus we have the cardiovascular nurse specialist, the diabetic nurse, the ostomy nurse, etc. On units where Primary Nursing is successfully implemented, a different delineation of nurse specialisation often emerges spontaneously.

Before implementing the system on an oncology unit, I assumed the nurses' area of clinical expertise was a combination of knowledge about the care of patients with cancer who were undergoing chemotherapy and radiation therapy. After successful implementation I learned that the truly unique contribution that the nurses developed was in the area of caring for dying patients. Because of nursing's unique continuous presence, it was logical and sensible for nurses to become expert in helping patients and their families experience death in a supportive, therapeutic atmosphere.

On an obstetrics unit, where I thought the nurses' area of expertise was post-partum care (breast feeding, bathing the baby and checking the episiotomy, etc.), I found that their real expertise lay in assisting patients to adjust to parenthood or enhancing their adjustment to the new family reality.

In other words, Primary Nursing, by focusing care on the person rather than on tasks, physicians, diseases or drugs, promotes a completely natural development of new definitions of clinical specialisation. Careful analyses of these new roles need to be pursued by scholars and academicians in order to delineate, define and test the usefulness of new groupings of knowledge for nursing curricula.

THE POWER OF KNOWLEDGE

The unique place of nursing in the health care delivery system is founded on the continuous knowledge that only the nurse can have of patient, participating as she does in all of the events that affect him 24 hours a day, seven days a week. For example, a nurse is present when the patient is operated on, is present at 2.00 am when he is consumed with apprehension about how his illness will affect his ability to provide for his family, is present at 7.00 am when the dreaded diagnosis is delivered by the family physician and is present when the patient reacts to the pain of a spinal tap or the removal of dressings covering disfiguring surgery. The Primary Nurse is present and available to the patient during that time of particular closeness, the morning bath. She is present to listen, to hear, to interact with the person hospitalised for treatment. In some cases, nurses can know the hospitalised patient better than members of his own family, at least in terms of his hospitalisation experience. The Primary Nursing system is designed to bring all of this knowledge together in one person who integrates and coordinates all aspects of the patient's care, making it possible to give care in a hospital that is as unified, personalised and humane as the private duty nursing of years gone by.

None of the other health disciplines involved in the treatment of the hospitalised person has access to this broad spectrum of knowledge. They must all depend on the eyes and ears of the nursing staff for much of the information they require.

This kind of knowledge is powerful. It has heretofore received inadequate attention, but the slowly emerging realisation of its value is helping to redefine the unique knowledge base upon which nursing as a profession can achieve a greater degree of autonomy. The Primary Nurse who appreciates and respects the importance of her knowledge will have a greater sense of self-esteem and the true worth of her contribution to patient care. As this sense develops and is recognised, both by herself and others, the Primary Nurse can claim her legitimate place beside other professionals and know the satisfaction of a dream finally achieved.

APPENDIX
COMMONLY ASKED QUESTIONS ABOUT PRIMARY NURSING ANSWERED WITH COMMON SENSE

DOES THE PRIMARY NURSE ALWAYS WORK THE DAY SHIFT?

No, not necessarily. Since the day shift is usually more heavily staffed then either evenings or nights, it stands to reason that the majority of Primary Nurses will be assigned to work days. Also, the day nurse has the greatest opportunity to maintain good communication links with the other members of the health team (most of whom, for some reason, also work only the day shift).

In hospitals where there is shift rotation, Primary Nurse/patient assignments will usually remain intact when a nurse rotates from days to evenings. The logic is that the nurse can continue to maintain a therapeutic relationship with the patient even though she is working evenings (the patient is awake and can communicate) and that the integrity of the relationship is very important. Admittedly, the Primary Nurse may have to compromise the direct communication element of the system, but that compromise is of secondary importance to the maintenance of the relationship. When a Primary Nurse rotates to nights, however, if she still has primary patients (she would usually not be assigned new patients prior to night rotation) they might well be reassigned to one of the day or evening nurses.

In hospitals which have permanent shift assignments, evening and night nurses can have Primary Nurse assignments, but their caseload is usually smaller than that of day nurses. The decision about which patients to assign to permanent evening and night nurses ought to focus on patient needs. Some patients seem to require the most sophisticated level of nursing on the 3 to 11 shift after family members go home. Other patients have trouble sleeping nights and require the most thoughtful attention on that tour of duty. These and other such considerations should be taken into account in making evening and night assignments. From a staffing standpoint it is seldom, if ever, necessary to assign the night nurse a Primary Nurse caseload; this type of assignment should be made when it makes sense for a particular patient, rather than as a routine.

A word about nurses who are not Primary Nurses. Special care must be taken to avoid the development of yet another second-class citizenship in nursing, this one between Primary Nurses and all other staff members. Those who are not Primary Nurses ought not to be made to feel that they are less worthy in any sense. The worth of a contribution must not be based on titles. A smoothly operating floor works only because of the contributions of all the staff working together—from new graduate to ward clerk, from nurses' aide to Primary Nurse. Individuals must be valued because of their contributions to the overall system; no one should feel diminished in stature because of Primary Nursing.

WHO SHOULD ASSIGN THE PATIENT? WHAT ABOUT THE IDEA OF NURSES SELECTING THEIR OWN PATIENTS?

The assignment of a Primary Nurse to a patient is usually made within 24 hours after admission. While the assignment decision is not usually difficult or time-consuming to make, it is complex, involving consideration of many factors. The head nurse as manager has ultimate responsibility for this function as a part of her overall duties of resource allocation. In many instances the Primary Nurse assignment decision becomes a matter of staff nurse decision making, which is based on clinical interests, workload, ability, needs of the patients, etc. *It doesn't matter* if the Primary Nurse assignment is made by the head nurse, a charge nurse, a specially designated staff nurse, or each Primary Nurse. The head nurse can choose to delegate this responsibility as long as the staff member designated uses good judgment. If problems of poor judgment arise, though, the head nurse has the ultimate responsibility for resolving them.

DOES THE PATIENT HAVE ANYTHING TO SAY ABOUT WHO HIS/HER PRIMARY NURSE IS?

Yes, an important factor in the Primary Nurse assignment is the patient's right to participate in the decision-making process. Since most nurses are not initially known by the newly admitted patients, participation at the point of admission is usually limited to patients who have been previously hospitalised on the unit. If at any time during a patient's hospitalisation he or she expresses the desire to change Primary Nurses, or expresses an inability to relate well with his Primary Nurse, reassignment should be made quickly and with impunity. Nurses frequently ask me how to handle the situation in which they do not get along with the patient they have been assigned. My answer is always that you should be able to request reassignment without its becoming an issue and the same is true when a patient does not get along with the nurse. Extreme care must be taken to ensure that a patient requesting reassignment to a different Primary Nurse is in no way punished or negatively treated by any of the staff. In any situation where the patient has an opportunity to know the staff members, such as small community hospitals or in cases where the patient is being rehospitalised, every effort should be made to permit the patient to choose his own Primary Nurse as long as his selection is therapeutically effective.

HOW DOES PRIMARY NURSING WORK FOR THE CHRONICALLY ILL PATIENT WHO IS HOSPITALISED FOR AN EXTENDED PERIOD OF TIME?

This question usually leads to a more widespread issue regarding nurse/patient assignments: What do you do if a nurse gets tired of a patient or is not, *for any reason*, getting along with him? Since the essence of Primary Nursing is the establishment of a therapeutic relationship, failure to achieve or maintain such a relationship is adequate justification for reassignment. This is a completely normal situation which should be handled without chastising either the patient or the nurse.

Chronically ill patients are not necessarily 'problem patients'. Many nurses find they offer an especially rewarding type of challenge. However, during long-term hospitalisation, two types of reassignment situations may occur. First, a Primary Nurse may need to be relieved of daily care activities once in a while. This should be done in a matter of fact manner. Second, a nurse may need to be relieved temporarily or permanently of her Primary Nurse responsibilities. This too should be accomplished in a matter of fact manner, making sure the patient understands the change without being made to feel rejected by the Primary Nurse.

DO ALL PATIENTS NEED A PRIMARY NURSE?

Yes. Rather than considering the question on a need basis, I prefer to answer on a 'right' basis. I believe all patients have a right to know who is making decisions regarding their nursing care and who is 'in charge' of it. When patients have the names of the responsible physician and the responsible nurse managing their cases, true accountability for hospital care can be established.

Because Primary Nursing is incredibly difficult to implement in settings where immature attitudes prevail, I do not feel it will be available to all patients in the foreseeable future. However, wherever the system is implemented, I believe all patients in that setting (hospital, or floor, or patient care division) have an equal right to know the names of the nurses responsible for their care. Thus, *I feel it is unfair and unwise to have some patients with a Primary Nurse and others without one in a single unit.*

HOW ABOUT A VERY SHORT-TERM PATIENT—ONE WHO IS HOSPITALISED JUST OVERNIGHT?

Since that patient will be receiving some nursing care during his short stay, I see no reason why he should not know the name of the nurse responsible for that care. Someone will be making some kind of decisions. The question is whether or not the patient need know who that person is when he is in so briefly, and the answer is still 'yes'. It may not be necessary to have a nursing care plan or discharge plan for the short-term patient, but Primary Nursing is visible responsibility for decision making, not the existence of elaborate care plans.

WHAT IS AN ASSOCIATE PRIMARY NURSE? SHOULD AN ASSOCIATE NURSE ALWAYS TAKE CARE OF THE SAME PRIMARY NURSE'S PATIENTS EACH DAY?

The words 'associate nurse' were originally used to describe the role of the staff member who took care of the patient when the Primary Nurse was off duty, and it is in this sense that I have used them. In some hospitals, however, the words have been used as a job description rather than a shift role assignment. I do not agree with the use of 'associate Primary Nurse' as a job title for many reasons, not the least of which is that it creates another level in an already too-many-layered hierarchy.

The system of Primary Nursing builds in continuity of care through the Primary Nurse who takes care of her own patient each shift she works and who leaves instructions for others to follow. Some hospitals have tried to enhance that continuity by maintaining continuity of the associate nurse/patient assignment. The logistics of accomplishing this are awkward but if it can be managed without inordinately complex planning then care must be taken to prevent excessive isolation among station personnel. In Primary Nursing staff members develop a much more profound knowledge of fewer patients, but it is still important that all staff members have at least a general idea of what is going on with all the patients. I find it helpful to think of Primary Nurse, associate Primary Nurse, or charge nurse as ad hoc role assignments any experienced registered nurse should be expected to be able to perform, rather than thinking of them as position titles. This increases the flexibility of utilisation of the staff. Then associate Primary Nurse assignments can be handled by different individuals depending on the circumstances on a shift. Continuity is maintained through the Primary Nurse's instructions.

WHAT IS THE ROLE OF THE CLINICAL SPECIALIST?

Without getting into the controversy about educational preparation, I will define clinical specialist as one who has a greater scope and breadth of clinical knowledge in a particular field than that of the average staff nurse. Using this definition, the contribution of the clinical specialist is made whenever a staff nurse is caring for a patient whose care needs require clinical knowledge at the specialist level. The Primary Nurse requests a consult from the specialist who makes an assessment and leaves recommendations. The Primary Nurse must be free to accept or reject these recommendations since she has superior knowledge of the total patient. If she decides to reject the specialist's recommendations she should be expected to be able to explain her rationale for doing so to the head nurse who is ultimately responsible for the quality of care administered to all the patients on the unit. The logical role then for clinical specialists in Primary Nursing is that of expert consultant. They can also make a significant contribution as Primary Nurses themselves for patients with extremely complex care requirements, or as co-Primary Nurses to back up a staff nurse in a complicated clinical situation. In addition, the clinical specialist ought to be available to teach nurses whatever they need to know in order to continue improving patient care.

SHOULD THE HEAD NURSE TAKE A PRIMARY NURSE ASSIGNMENT?

It doesn't matter. Many head nurses have found after implementing this system that they have time to manage a small caseload, usually one or two patients. By doing so, they can share in the dynamic rewards of being a nurse for a sick person and can also provide a powerful role model. Sometimes head nurses prefer to be associate Primary Nurses and use this opportunity to strengthen a new nurse's knowledge base, assess her learning, and so on. Some head nurses function as a Primary Nurse at times, and as an associate at others and as neither when their head nurse responsibilities require their full attention. However, some head nurses decide never to take a patient assignment, either as associate or as Primary Nurse. If they are able to establish an effective teacher/clinician/leader role using other techniques, having caseloads of their own is not vitally important.

REFERENCES

1. This and other quotations in this chapter are taken from the student records of the Connecticut Training School, New Haven, for the years 1890 to 1910.
2. Kramer, M. *Reality Shock*. St Louis: Mosby, 1974.
3. Gelinas, A. *Nursing and Nursing Education*. New York: The Commonwealth Fund, 1946, p. 9.
4. Brown, EL. *Nursing for the Future*. New York: Russell Sage Foundation, 1944.
5. *Towards Quality in Nursing—Report of the Surgeon General's Consultant Group in Nursing*. Washington, DC: United States Public Health Service, 1963. p. 15.
6. Ibid.
7. Kramer, ibid.
8. American Nursing Association, Committee on Education. ANA's first position paper on education for nursing, *Am J. Nurs.* 65:106, 1965.
9. Aydelotte, MK and Tever, ME *An Investigation of the Relation Between Nursing Activity and Patient Welfare*. Iowa City: State University of Iowa, 1960.
10. United States Public Health Service, Division of Nursing. *How to Study Activities on a Patient Unit* (rev. ed.). Washington, DC: US Government Printing Office (PHS Publication No. 570), 1964.
11. Ibid.
12. Personal communication by group of nurses doing Primary Nursing at Yale-New Haven Hospital interviewed by author during 1979.
13. Ibid.
14. Barrett, J. *Word Management and Teaching*. London: Appleton-Century-Crofts, 1949.
15. Goodman, P. *People or Personnel: Decentralizing and the Mixed System*. Toronto: Random House, 1965.
16. Vaillot, Sister Madeline Clemence. Existentialism: A philosophy of commitment, *Am. J. Nurs.* 66:38, 1966.

INDEX

Academic degrees, 33–34
Accountability, 4, 19, 21, 23, 51, 55, 56
Adaptability, 7–8
Administrative structure, systems, 57, 62
  organisational theory, 55
Administrators, hospital, 15, 18
Administrators, nurse, 15, 16, 18
Advisory council, 61, 63
Alumnae Associations, 3, 5
American Nurses Association, 5, 16
  1965 Position Paper, 32
American Red Cross, 12
Associate degree programmes, 16
Associate Primary Nurses, 34, 73–4
Authority, 17
  commensurate with responsibility, 38, 56,
    61
  natural levels of, 56–7
Autonomy, 70
Auxiliary personnel, 12, 14, 19
Aydelotte, Myrtle Kitchel, 18

Baccalaureate programmes, nurses, 16, 32,
  33
Barrett, Jean, 38
Boards of registry, 3–5
Brown, Esther Lucille, 13
Budgets, 39
Bureaucracies, 1, 4, 10, 12, 31, 56, 65

Cadet Corps, 12
Care plans, 21–3, 27, 28, 32, 51–3, 73
  modifications in, 34, 45
Case load, 67, 68, 71
Case method, 9, 12, 19, 26, 29, 44, 48
Charge nurse, 46, 72, 74
Clinical specialist, 74
Communication, 19, 71

complex channels of, 20–1
direct channels of, 30
with other members of the health team,
  31
with patients, 31
patterns, 45–7
skills, 47, 52
at station level, 30
Community health education, 3
Consensus, 48–9
Continuity of nursing care, 22, 30, 49, 74
Cost containment, 38–9

Data collection, 44, 59–60
Day shift, 71
Decision making, decision-making
  authority 2, 26, 30, 32, 37, 40, 48, 50,
    59, 66–8
  allocation of, 56
  autonomy, 3
  decentralised, 27, 39, 40, 55
  participation in, 41
  responsibility for, 26, 56
  teaching of, 66–7
Delegated medical tasks (DMT), 17
Depression of 1929, 11
Deprofessionalisation of nursing practice, 2,
  10
Diploma programmes, 16
Director of nursing, 57, 61, 62, 63
Discharge planning, 28, 45, 62, 73

Education, 2, 8, 13, 15–16, 68
  clinician/teacher method, 66
  level of, 32–3
  reintegration with service, 66
Educational resources, 51, 53, 61, 65
Evaluation, 4, 53–4